# Poverty, Welfare and the Disciplinary State

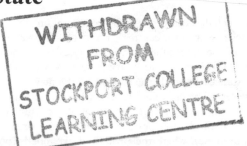

*Poverty, Welfare and the Disciplinary State* argues that the social-democratic welfare state which came into being in Britain after the second world war should now be seen as a brief departure from a more ruthless form of social policy that has traditionally characterised the state's response to some of the poorest people in society. The book argues that since 1979 there has been a new ruthlessness in social policy which has been influential in the creation of what it describes as the disciplinary state, which is evident in a number of advanced capitalist societies and shows no sign of being reined back. In this context the book examines such issues as:

- the current dynamics of poverty in Britain, drawing on similar developments in Europe and the US
- the major areas of social policy within which this abandonment and demonisation of the poor is taking place
- the historical antecedents to this relationship between the state and the poor
- the creation and expansion of a 'welfare' state that characterised the era of social democracy until the mid-1970s and, from the point of view of the poor, was limited and conditional
- the ideology and organisation of the new right and of New Labour
- the new terrain on which the struggle over the future of welfare and social policy must take place.

It will appeal to all students of social policy, social work and sociology.

**Chris Jones** is Professor of Social Policy and Social Work at Liverpool University; **Tony Novak** is Lecturer in Social Policy also at Liverpool University.

114781

# The State of Welfare
## Edited by Mary Langan

Nearly half a century after its post-war consolidation, the British welfare state is once again at the centre of political controversy. After a decade in which the role of the state in the provision of welfare was steadily reduced in favour of the private, voluntary and informal sectors, with relatively little public debate or resistance, the further extension of the new mixed economy of welfare in the spheres of health and education became a major political issue in the early 1990s. At the same time the impact of deepening recession has begun to expose some of the deficiencies of market forces in areas such as housing and income maintenance, where their role had expanded dramatically during the 1980s. *The State of Welfare* provides a forum for continuing the debate about the services we need as we enter the twenty-first century.

Titles of related interest also in *The State of Welfare* series:

**Taking Child Abuse Seriously**
*The Violence Against Children Study Group*

**Women, Oppression and Social Work**
*Edited by Mary Langan and Lesley Day*

**Managing Poverty: The Limits of Social Assistance**
*Carol Walker*

**Towards a Post-Fordist Welfare State?**
*Roger Burrows and Brian Loader*

**Working with Men: Feminism and Social Work**
*Edited by Kate Cavanagh and Viviene E. Cree*

**Social Theory, Social Change and Social Work**
*Edited by Nigel Parton*

**Working for Equality in Health**
*Edited by Paul Bywaters and Eileen McLeod*

**Social Action for Children and Families**
*Edited by Crescy Cannan and Chris Warren*

**Child Protection and Family Support**
*Nigel Parton*

**Social Work and Child Abuse**
*David Merrick*

**Towards a Classless Society?**
*Edited by Helen Jones*

# Poverty, Welfare and the Disciplinary State

**Chris Jones and Tony Novak**

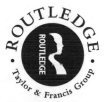

London and New York

First published 1999
by Routledge
11 New Fetter Lane, London EC4P 4EE

Simultaneously published in the USA and Canada
by Routledge
29 West 35th Street, New York, NY 10001

© 1999 Chris Jones and Tony Novak

Typeset in Times by
M Rules
Printed and bound in Great Britain by
TJ International Ltd, Padstow, Cornwall

*British Library Cataloguing in Publication Data*
A catalogue record for this book is available from the British
Library

*Library of Congress Cataloging in Publication Data*
A record for this book has been requested

ISBN 0 415 18289 1 (hbk)
ISBN 0 415 18290 5 (pbk)

# Contents

# Series editor's preface

State welfare policies reflect changing perceptions of key sources of social instability. In the first half of the twentieth century – from Bismarck to Beveridge – the welfare state emerged as a set of policies and institutions which were, in the main, a response to the 'problem of labour', the threat of class conflict. The major objective was to contain and integrate the labour movement. In the post-war decades, as this threat receded, the welfare state became consolidated as a major employer and provider of a wide range of services and benefits to every section of society. Indeed it increasingly became the focus of blame for economic decline and was condemned for its inefficiency and ineffectiveness.

Since the end of the Cold War the major fear of capitalist societies is no longer class conflict but the socially disintegrative consequences of the system itself. A heightened awareness of the manifestations of social instability – including unemployment and homelessness, delinquency, drug abuse and crime, divorce, single parenthood and child abuse – reflects deep-seated apprehensions about the future of modern society.

The role of state social policy in the Clinton–Blair era is to restrain and regulate the destructive effects of market forces symbolised by the Reagan–Thatcher years. On both sides of the Atlantic governments have rejected the old polarities of left and right, the goals of both comprehensive state intervention and rampant free-market individualism. In its pursuit of a 'third way' the New Labour government which came to power in Britain in May 1997 has sought to define a new role for government at a time when politics has largely retreated from its traditional concerns about the nature and direction of society.

For Tony Blair, the third way is 'based on values, not on outdated ideology' (*The Times*, 25 July 1998). Its starting point is the conviction that people should adjust to the diminished possibilities offered by a society in which change for the better seems no longer very feasible. This is how Anthony Giddens, director of the London School of

Economics and a key intellectual influence on New Labour, puts it: 'In a situation where change has long ceased to be all progress, if it ever was, and where progress has become eminently disputable, the preservation and renewal of tradition, as well as of environmental resources, take on a particular urgency' (Giddens 1994: 49).

What are the values of the third way? According to Tony Blair, the people of Middle England 'distrust heavy ideology' but want 'security and stability'; they 'want to refashion the bonds of community life' and 'although they believe in the market economy, they do not believe that the only values that matter are those of the market place' (*The Times*, 25 July 1998). The values of the third way reflect and shape a traditional and conservative response to the dynamic and unpredictable world of the late 1990s.

The view expressed by Michael Jacobs (1998), a leading participant in the revived Fabian Society, that 'we live in a strongly individualised society which is falling apart' is widely shared. For him, 'the fundamental principle' of the third way is 'to balance the autonomous demands of the individual with the need for social cohesion or "community"'. A key New Labour concept that follows from this preoccupation with community is that of 'social exclusion'. Proclaimed the government's 'most important innovation' when it was announced in August 1997, the 'social-exclusion unit' is at the heart of New Labour's flagship social-policy initiative – the 'welfare-to-work' programme. The preoccupation with 'social exclusion' indicates a concern about tendencies towards fragmentation in society and a self-conscious commitment to policies which seek to integrate atomised individuals and thus to enhance social cohesion.

The popularity of the concept of social exclusion reflects a striking tendency to aggregate diverse issues so as to imply a common origin. The concept of social exclusion legitimises the moralising dynamic of New Labour. Initiatives such as 'welfare to work', targeting the young unemployed and single mothers, emphasise individual responsibility. Duties – to work, to save, to adopt a healthy lifestyle, to do homework, to 'parent' in the approved manner – are the common themes of New Labour social policy; obligations take precedence over rights.

Though the concept of social exclusion targets a smaller section of society than earlier categories such as 'the poor' or 'the underclass', it does so in a way which does imply a societal responsibility for the problems of fragmentation, as well as indicating a concern to draw people back – from truancy, sleeping rough, delinquency and drugs, etc. – into the mainstream of society. Yet New Labour's sympathy for the excluded only extends as far as the provision of voluntary work and training schemes, parenting classes and drug rehabilitation programmes. The socially excluded are no longer allowed to be the passive recipients of benefits; they are obliged to participate in their moral reintegration. Those who refuse to subject themselves to these apparently benign forms of regulation may soon find themselves the target of more coercive interventions.

There is a third feature of New Labour's third way. The very novelty of New Labour initiatives necessitates the appointment of new person-nel and the creation of new institutions to overcome the inertia of the established structures of central and local government. To emphasise the importance of its drugs policy the government has created the new office of Drugs Commissioner – 'Tsar' – and prefers to implement the policy through a plethora of voluntary organisations, rather than through traditional channels. Health action zones, education action zones and employment action zones are the chosen vehicles for policy innovation in their respective areas. At higher levels of government, semi-detached special policy units, think tanks and quangos play an increasingly impor-tant role.

*The State of Welfare* aims to provide a critical assessment of social policy in the new millennium. The series will consider the new and emerging third-way welfare policies and practices and the way these are shaped by wider social and economic changes. Globalisation, the emergence of post-industrial society, the transformation of work, demo-graphic shifts and changes in gender roles and family structures all have major consequences for patterns of welfare provision.

Social policy will also be affected by the demands of social move-ments – women, minority ethnic groups, disabled people, as well as groups concerned with sexuality or the environment. *The State of Welfare* will examine these influences when analysing welfare practices in the first decade of the new millennium.

Mary Langan<br>February 1999

## References

Giddens, A. (1994) *Beyond Left and Right: The Future of Radical Politics.* Cambridge: Polity.

Jacobs, M. (1998) *The Third Way*. London: The Fabian Society.

# Preface

This has been a difficult book to complete, and the story it tells about the mounting toll of poverty and inequality in contemporary Britain is in many ways unfinished. Rarely does a day pass without some news report detailing yet another dimension of the suffering and indignity which many millions in our society face, or yet another twist of the screw of a government policy that contributes to rather than alleviates this situation. What began as an attempt to make sense of eighteen years of political domination in Britain by avowedly right-wing governments, intent upon celebrating inequality and dismissing poverty as irrelevant, has also had to take account, since 1997, of a new political party in power. That this has not caused us to change our analysis, while a matter of deep disappointment, also confirms the scale of the problem and indicates how much more still needs to be done.

Many things have driven us to write this book. The most obvious has been the need to try to describe and understand what has been going on in a society that has witnessed such massive reversals in fortune for such a large number of people in such a relatively short period of time. In this we have also been in part motivated by disappointment with a number of academic accounts and studies; while these are sometimes useful in providing data which set out the scale of the changes that have taken place, they too often fail to capture the human catastrophes that are the reality behind the facts and figures they present. Poverty and inequality are amongst the most fundamental human-rights abuses in the world today. They distort, corrode and destroy people's lives. They condemn vast numbers to intolerable conditions which are neither acceptable nor necessary in a world which has the capacity to provide every single person with the means of a decent, human existence. That this potential is not realised is not some inevitable mystery of nature, but rather a consequence of human agency. It need not be.

The primary inspiration for our task has been the courage, determination and struggle of those who have borne the brunt of the economic, political and ideological onslaught that has characterised this new and more brutal phase of capitalist development. Their endurance is a testament to the resilience and generosity of the human spirit. We would also acknowledge the contribution to our work of those investigative journalists and writers, such as Nick Davies, John Pilger, David Rose, Bea Campbell, and others, and of campaigners and activists like Bob Holman, who have provided us with insights into the human dimensions of poverty and the brutality and indignity which are also part of the condition of poverty in contemporary society. We do not personally know any of these writers, but their work has been of great importance to us and we thank them. We would also like to acknowledge the work of Richard Wilkinson and Nancy Hollander, both of whom have explored the devastation caused to the well-being of the poor by the abusive ideologies and practices which accompany the management and control of poverty in many parts of the world. We also owe a considerable debt to a number of organisations campaigning over issues such as low pay and unemployment, and in particular to the Child Poverty Action Group (CPAG), which for over thirty years has doggedly documented and publicised the shifting terrain of poverty.

It is not just the massive increase in poverty that has concerned us, but the ways in which the ruling elites in Britain and elsewhere have come to denigrate the poor. They appear to have no shame in dismissing the victims and casualties of an increasingly harsh, not to say triumphalist, economic system as 'losers' and as various debased forms of 'low life' now encapsulated in their depiction as an 'underclass'. Nor do they hesitate to adopt policies which so clearly increase their misery. These are ugly and frightening developments. As the history of the twentieth century should remind us, whether in fascist Germany or contemporary Yugoslavia, such depictions of human beings are one of the key features of genocide and barbarism. They are also used to justify and legitimate new social arrangements which contribute towards an increasingly authoritarian society: developments which, while focused on some, have the capacity to be extended to many. Again, we would like to acknowledge the work of those involved in publications such as *Statewatch*, *CARF* (Campaign Against Racism and Fascism) and *Race and Class*, who have so diligently investigated and reported on these developments. They deserve our recognition and much wider attention.

Finally, to the book itself. Even in its never-to-be-finished state we

have attempted to both describe and explain some of these developments. Like all authors we hope that readers will engage with the book
as a whole, but recognise that many will only dip into its various pages.
So, as a guide, the book is structured as follows. In Chapter 1 we set out
a number of themes which we subsequently develop in later chapters
through an exploration of what is involved in the contemporary redefinition of the poor as an 'underclass'. In this, as in the rest of the book,
we are also concerned to establish historical continuities as well as new
developments. Chapter 2 moves on to consider some of the key factors
contributing to the deepening of poverty and social polarisation, especially marked in Britain and the USA, where an unleashing of market
forces in combination with a reduction of state support for those who
need it have had such devastating consequences. In Chapter 3 we move
from looking at the material conditions of poverty to its social relationships, which are equally if not more important in determining what
it means to be poor. Here we focus on other ways in which the poor in
general and some of the poorest in particular are abused, principally at
the hands of state agencies. Chapter 4 offers an historical analysis of
capitalism and social reform to reveal how Adam Smith's vile maxim of
the masters – all for us and nothing for the rest – remains as valid today
as when it was first promulgated two centuries ago. In Chapter 5 we try
to make sense of what is happening within the state as it seeks to
manage and secure a deeply divided society. Finally in Chapter 6 we
explore current political developments, especially in the light of the
election of a Labour government in Britain in 1997. Needless to say,
this chapter is the most speculative, although after eighteen months we
have to conclude that little has changed. While it gives us no joy to say
so, it rather confirms the criticism made 150 years ago by the British
working-class co-operative movement of parliamentary reform that
'merely changed the form of government without changing the form of
society'.

Chris Jones and Tony Novak
October 1998

# 1   Redefining the poor

In February 1993, following the killing of 2-year-old Jamie Bulger by two young children, John Major, the British Prime Minister, urged the country 'to condemn a little more and to understand a little less'. His comments came in the wake of a mass of media reports and scrutiny that had portrayed this tragic but rare and isolated event as symptomatic of a much wider and deep-rooted malaise within British society, most especially amongst the working-class poor. Over the following days and weeks pages of newsprint and television documentaries represented the event as a defining moment in British social and cultural life: as symbolising a fundamental breakdown of moral order, reflected not only in the apparently senseless death of a young child, but also in a fear of rising crime in general, in rioting and other social disturbances on the part of young people, and, linked to these, high levels of dependency on state benefits and the disintegration of the family and its mechanisms of order and control within poor working-class communities. In its lead editorial of 28 February 1993, the *Sunday Times*, which had long campaigned on these issues, encapsulated this concern in a scathing attack on a 'popular culture' which, it argued, had come to despise and undermine the traditional nuclear family. Laying the blame firmly at the feet of the 'British intelligentsia', it went on:

> Now the nation is having to deal with the consequences of this *trahison des clercs* in the form of soaring crime, increasing squalor, widespread welfare dependency, the spread of the yob culture and crumbling communities . . . It is becoming increasingly clear to all but the most blinkered of social scientists that the disintegration of the nuclear family is the principal source of so much social unrest and misery. The creation of an urban underclass, on the margins of society but doing great damage to itself and the rest of us, is directly linked to the rapid rise in illegitimacy . . . The past two

decades have witnessed the growth of whole communities in which the dominant family structure is the single-parent mother on welfare, whose male offspring are already immersed in a criminal culture by the time they are teenagers and whose daughters are destined to follow in the family tradition of unmarried teenage mothers. It is not just a question of a few families without fathers; it is a matter of whole communities with barely a single worthwhile male role-model. No wonder the youths of the underclass are uncontrollable by the time (sometimes before) they are teenagers . . . In communities without fathers, the overwhelming evidence is that youngsters begin by running wild and end up running foul of the law.

*(Sunday Times* 28 February 1993)

The 'overwhelming evidence' for such an argument was, as we shall see, by no means so clear-cut. But this was not really the point. The Bulger tragedy allowed the media, politicians and a range of other commentators to portray Britain as in a state of terminal moral decline. At the heart of this decline, it was argued, lay the erosion of 'family values', of respect for the law and for authority, and the weakening of the work ethic – the values that had made Britain 'Great'. It was not, as we shall see, a new concern; nor did the fact that it harked back to a mythical golden age, or greatly exaggerated and distorted the social changes that had indeed occurred over the previous decades, diminish the force of its argument. On the contrary, it fed into a way of looking at British society, and at the poor and the most marginalised in particular, that was to replace reality, objectivity and understanding with myth, dogma and condemnation. In a rare exception to the hysteria which the news media in particular whipped up, Neil Ascherson, writing in the *Independent on Sunday*, warned of the need to look more closely at what was going on:

We are going through a period of monstrously artificial media uproars – stories which are exaggerated and inflated into 'issues' supposed to reveal this or that sickness of our society . . . The trick in such spasms of provoked anxiety is to look in the opposite direction. Who exactly wants the British public to understand less and condemn more? Who is encouraging us to demonise sections of our society as if they had been infiltrated by aliens? . . . What is this spectacle really about? It is about the grand British engineering project of the 1990s – the construction of the Underclass. Much of the preparatory work has already been done. Unemployment has passed three million . . . welfare payments have been reduced, inequality has been drastically increased, and an imaginative programme for poverty creation is on the way to completion. What remains, in the second phase, is to shift the whole bottom third of British society to these new foundations, by establishing that poverty, combined with idleness and savagery, is its natural and incurable condition.

(*Independent on Sunday* 28 February 1993)

Holding the poor responsible for their poverty has been a constant ever since the word – and the poor themselves – first appeared in the Middle Ages. But it has been tempered, and at times over-ridden, by different and competing explanations such as injustice, oppression, exploitation, misfortune or the inadequacy of social support that have offered alternative understandings and solutions. With the emergence of the concept of the poor as an 'underclass' over the past decade the victim-blaming ideology of poverty has returned with a vengeance. In this new description or construction of the poor there is little if any recognition of the devastating structural changes that have reshaped British society over the past twenty years: the failure of the labour market and the re-emergence of mass and long-term unemployment, the withdrawal of welfare services, the widening gap between rich and poor, or the effects of prolonged poverty on individuals, families and communities. On the contrary, according to Charles Murray, a member of the American Enterprise Institute, the right-wing US think tank whose book *Losing Ground* has been credited with providing the 'blueprint for the Reagan administration's war on welfare' (McCrate and Smith 1998: 64), members of the 'underclass' are 'defined by their behaviour' (Murray 1990: 1). In the late 1980s Murray was sponsored by the *Sunday Times* to spend a year in Britain in order to study 'the emerging British underclass'. As he himself put it 'I arrived in Britain earlier this year, a visitor from a plague area come to see whether the disease is spreading' (Murray 1990: 3). His conclusions predictably were that at the core of the poverty problem in Britain were a group of people identified by their abnormal and amoral values and their wilful rejection of the norms of the society around them: 'Britain has a growing population of working-aged, healthy people who live in a different world from other Britons, who are raising their children to live in it, and whose values are now contaminating the life of entire neighbourhoods' (Murray 1990: 4).

This image of a 'different world' is a recurring theme in such depictions of the poor, at the same time both alien and threatening. In 1983 the Metropolitan Police Commissioner spoke of 'what many commentators refer to as "the underclass" – a class that is beneath the working class' that was to be found 'where unemployed youths – often black youths – congregate . . . They equate closely with the criminal rookeries of Dickensian London' (cited Campbell 1993: 108). The drawing of the historical parallel is significant. As John Macnicol has argued:

> The concept of an inter-generational underclass displaying a high concentration of social problems – remaining outwith the boundaries of citizenship, alienated from cultural norms and stubbornly impervious to the normal incentives of the market, social work intervention or state welfare – has been reconstructed periodically over at least the past one hundred years, and while there have been important shifts of emphasis between each of these reconstructions, there have also been striking continuities. Underclass stereotypes have always been a part of the discourse on poverty in advanced industrial societies.
>
> (Macnicol 1987: 296)

While something of an historical constant, such stereotypes have differed significantly over time, both in their dominance over other explanations and, importantly, in the extent to which they have seen the poor as capable of escaping their fate. In the 1960s and 1970s poverty, despite its persistence, was widely seen as something that, with proper intervention, could be eradicated. By the 1990s poverty has become seen, when it is mentioned at all, as largely inevitable, as the consequence of the actions or failures on the part of poor people themselves, and something which not even economic growth can solve. In general such pessimistic and negative constructions of the poor have tended to be most prevalent and powerful, and the view of their innate defects most rigid, at times of high levels of poverty and unemployment. So it was in the 1830s and the 1880s, as well as in the 1930s and now in the fourth great cyclical depression to afflict modern capitalism. This relationship between the labour market and dominant conceptions of poverty has always been significant in shaping state policies and practices. It is when the system is most under threat – when its claim to equality and fairness is most visibly denied by the distress and unfairness it manifestly creates – that poor people have been subject to the most criticism and attack. In this process both the reality and the consequences of poverty are denied, and the lives of the poor both disparaged and distorted. Thus according to David Hunt, Employment Secretary in the Conservative government in 1994:

It is often said that poverty and unemployment create crime. In my experience the converse is true . . . Some of the so-called cultures springing up in our country reject all decency and civilised values – the cultures of the housebreaker, the hippy and the hoodlum. The bulk of thieving today of course has nothing to do with poverty. It is the result of wickedness and greed.

(*Guardian* 21 March 1994)

At the end of the twentieth century when, particularly in Britain and the USA, the market economy has once again come to be celebrated as the most efficient, indeed the only possible, basis for economic and social life, it is no accident that there has been a return to harsh and brutalising depictions of those who are its greatest victims. With the collapse of communism, capitalism is triumphant, its ravages inflicted on a global scale. Holding the poor responsible for their own fate undermines the anger that poverty and inequality provoke while removing blame from the system that is responsible. Instead, the poor are seen as an expensive 'burden' on society, for whom the 'average taxpayer' supposedly has little sympathy, especially when depicted as welfare 'scroungers', homeless, criminals and drug addicts. As David Blunkett, later to become Secretary of State for Education in New Labour's government, put it, 'those committed to a new twenty-first century welfare state have to cease paternalistic and well-meaning indulgence of thuggery, noise, nuisance and anti-social behaviour' (*Independent* 28 February 1993). Just as the provision of welfare services is seen as encouraging their dependency, so its removal is justified as both reducing the cost and halting the supply of their numbers. The result is increasing distress and further poverty. But although, from the point of view of contemporary capitalism, the so-called 'underclass' are deemed to be surplus to current and future economic projections, in reality, as we shall see, their demonisation fulfils an essential economic and social purpose.

## Class and continuity

Punitive and negative images of the poor are deeply sedimented, historically, within British society. These images reflect not only the periodic reconstruction of the poor as morally degenerate and culpable, but also a more widespread, deep-rooted and long-standing antagonism that has characterised social and class relationships in Britain. These divisions, remarked upon by many commentators, especially from abroad, who see in Britain, and in England in particular, an entrenched divide between 'us' and 'them' and a culture and set of institutions that reflect, embody and maintain this, are in part the product of Britain's long historical experience of capitalism. The first country to create an industrial working class, it was some 200 years ago a society polarised into waged workers on the one hand, and an industrial, financial and landed aristocratic elite on the other to an extent unparalleled in any other country, some even to this day. Unlike in the rest of continental Europe, the independent peasantry in Britain was long ago eliminated, its transformation into a class of dependent wage workers achieved by a process of attrition and violence over many centuries before then. For the most part it was a very bloody history, and the scars still remain.

The fact also that the ruling class in Britain has remained in power, if not without challenge, then at least without overthrow, throughout this process has contributed to its sense of confidence and arrogance, as well as giving it its own historical experience of rule to draw upon. The British ruling class has proved, more than most others, eminently adaptable. It has throughout its history been more than prepared to use violence to defend its position and power, but it has also learned, when violence is not enough, to accommodate the challenges that have faced it. Thus the aristocratic order in Britain largely survived the challenge posed by the rise of capitalism, allying itself to the interests of the new bourgeoisie, where elsewhere it was overthrown. The British establishment – that curious mixture of wealth, power, tradition, church and state – has maintained its privilege through turbulence and challenge. The 'lower orders' have by and large been kept in their place; and the ruling class has maintained its continuity, buttressed by pomp and ceremony.

Allied to this has been a viciousness, admittedly present amongst ruling classes in many parts of the world, whereby simply to make money has never been enough. British capitalism has been fêted for the benevolence and humanitarianism of some of its owners: its enlightened employers such as Robert Owen and its social reformers and philanthropists. The more common reality is very different: Britain as the world leader in the inhuman slave trade, from which the former wealth of cities like Liverpool was made, its employers ruthless and determined, and its philanthropy, to coin a phrase, 'as cold as charity'. It is a history of contempt on the part of the ruling class towards those who work to maintain them in place.

If the British ruling class has viewed the poor in general with contempt, policy towards the poorest, especially those who could not or would not find work, has verged on hysteria and hatred. During the

Middle Ages the poor were, quite literally, branded as rogues and vagabonds, subjected to whippings and, ultimately, death as penalty for their fate. The callousness with which many mine and factory owners treated men, women and children during the course of the industrial revolution – treating their animals better than their workers – prompted international comment and even revulsion amongst a minority of the British establishment itself. It is a telling indication that Britain's elite formed a Royal Society for the Protection of Animals before it formed a similar organisation for the protection of children. During the nineteenth century the British state perfected what it saw as the ultimate policy for dealing with poverty – a national system of deterrent workhouses designed to instil terror in the minds of anyone in need of assistance. By the end of that century, faced with the outbreak of mass unemployment and rising poverty during the first great depression, the poor – or at least the poorest – were again to be redefined along familiar lines. Thus Charles Booth, one of Britain's most noted social investigators, wrote of those who 'from shiftlessness, helplessness, idleness or drink are inevitably poor . . . a deposit of those who from mental, moral and physical reasons are incapable of better work' (Booth 1904: 44). Seen as 'perhaps incapable of improvement' this 'residuum', as it came widely to be called, was, like today's 'underclass', to be subjected to increasingly punitive control and containment.

As in the second great depression of the 1930s, or indeed that of the 1980s, the able-bodied unemployed at the end of the nineteenth century were to be made a particular target. But the challenge of poverty as faced by politicians and reformers was to prevent its growth from becoming an issue of further working-class identification and mobilisation. In a context where, for most of the nineteenth century, poverty had been seen as an inescapable and necessary feature of working-class life, this required a redefinition of poverty that would demarcate 'the poor' from the rest of the working class. This was to be the lasting and ultimately limiting achievement of social investigators and reformers such as Charles Booth and Seebohm Rowntree.

Once separated, the poor were to be subject to further classification. The concept of the residuum – like that of the present-day 'underclass' – similarly defined a section of the poor not so much by their poverty as by their behaviour and morality. Earlier distinctions between the deserving and undeserving poor based on their ability to work were replaced with one based not on ability but on attitudes to work and self-reliance. Those deemed undeserving of state help were to be left to rot in the workhouse.

This punitive treatment of the residuum at the end of the nineteenth century was further influenced by the emerging 'science' of Social Darwinism and eugenics. The view that genetics and biology provided explanations of human behaviour in general, and of the behaviour of the poor in particular, was to an extent discredited by the later experience of fascism, although its continuation in state policy, most notably in perceptions of and policies and practice towards black, mentally ill and disabled people, indicates that it was never far from the surface (see for example Oliver and Barnes (1998) with respect to disabled people). Its resurgence as a respectable area of intellectual inquiry in the 1990s, as in Charles Murray's *The Bell Curve* (Hernstein and Murray 1994), or as the basis for 'experiments' such as the American Federal Violence Initiative to identify 100,000 inner-city children whose 'biochemical and genetic defects will make them prone to violence in later life' (*Guardian* 13 March 1995), serves to rationalise and individualise social distress. The violence that is a consequence of poverty, the rage and frustration that can lead people to destroy their own relationships and communities, is obscured under pseudo-scientific explanations that reveal the extremes of a view of the poor as a group that is qualitatively different and incapable of integration into normal society. It does not require too great a grasp of human history to realise that once groups of the population are defined as less than human this provides legitimation for policies of neglect and other more ruthless interventions and treatment (Scheper-Hughes 1997: 20).

During the second great depression of the 1920s and 1930s, the 'residuum' was to be reconstituted as 'the social problem group', with a sharply increased focus on its genetic inheritability. The 1929 Wood Report on Mental Deficiency thus characterised mental deficiency as symptomatic of and at the core of the wider problem of the poor:

> If we are to prevent the racial disaster of mental deficiency, we must deal not merely with mentally defective persons, but with the whole subnormal group from which the majority of them come . . . [This] would include a much larger proportion of insane persons, epileptics, paupers, criminals (especially recidivists), unemployables, habitual slum dwellers, prostitutes, inebriates and other social inefficients . . . The overwhelming majority of the families thus collected will belong to that section of the community which we propose to term the 'social problem' or 'subnormal' group. This group comprises approximately 10% in the social scale of most communities.
>
> (cited Macnicol 1987: 297 and 302)

These historical parallels are points to which we shall return a number of times in this book, for they point to both the limited repertoire and the recurrent themes within which capitalist societies deal with the enduring problem of poverty. These continuities are also important in that they provide legacies of ideas and understandings which often with relative ease can be drawn upon and revamped with considerable impact and influence.

Another parallel to which we will frequently refer is what might be termed the 'transatlantic connection'. Capitalism is both a global phenomenon and, in its particularity, an experience which is unique to the history, culture and formation of individual societies. There is in effect a number of different capitalisms, but within these both Britain and the USA share a great deal in common. In her account of family and children's policies in rich nations, Hewlett (1993) draws attention to the distinctive meanness of Anglo-American capitalism when compared with Japan and most of continental western Europe. They are both countries in which the family is left largely to struggle on its own, where children are to be 'seen and not heard'. Her compelling and convincing analysis in this one area of social policy reinforces Chomsky's (1993) account of the development of capitalism since the Columbian conquest of America. In this longer and more ambitious project, Chomsky presents a detailed indictment of the peculiar ruthlessness which characterised Anglo-American capitalism. For the purpose of our analysis, this is significantly so in terms of the ways that the state in both societies has responded to poverty. In recent years, from the first electoral triumphs and bastions of new right government under Thatcher and Reagan, through to the continuing 'special relationship' between their successors, Clinton and Blair, the two countries have increasingly converged, and continue to learn much from each other, in their definitions of social problems and the construction of their social policies. The reconstitution at least of certain sections of the poor as an 'underclass' is one such example of this transatlantic connection. It is a concept which in its barbarism is true to the special ruthlessness of Anglo-American capitalism and finds little resonance in other comparable advanced capitalist societies.

In the USA the idea of an 'underclass' has been used extensively since the 1960s to portray in particular the situation of the black American poor. Indeed, as a number of commentators have pointed out, the term has become synonymous with – and often used as a coded reference to – 'race'. The failure of most African-Americans to climb the ladder of opportunity has been a feature of American society since its origins. From the days of slavery, through waves of European and more latterly Hispanic and far eastern migration of labour to feed the requirements of the world's most powerful economy, African-Americans have remained at the bottom of the heap.

Justification of this has readily adopted racist stereotypes – from the paternalistic images in slavery of black people as helpless children, though still to be bought and sold as objects, through the official definition in the post-emancipation Constitution of the USA of black people as two-thirds of a human being, to the modern counterpart of the black underclass. In its modern form, African-American poverty is described as the consequence of the breakdown and failure of the black family, the inability, or more commonly the refusal, of African-American males to adopt the capitalist work ethic, and the absence of norms within the black community that engender respect for property, law and order. More recently still, the genetic disposition of African-Americans to poverty that characterised much discussion prior to the second world war has returned to seal the fate of the poor as an inescapable product of biology.

In this way, the poor who are seen to constitute an 'underclass' are viewed as fundamentally different from the rest of the population. Indeed, it was, according to Murray, the blurring of this distinction during the 'intellectual reformation' of the 1960s that laid part of the ground for its future growth:

> Henceforth the poor were to be homogenised. The only difference between poor people and everyone else, we were told, was that the poor had less money. More importantly, the poor were all alike . . . Poor people, *all* poor people, were equally victims, and would be equally successful if only society gave them a fair shake.
>
> (Murray 1990: 2)

It is the redrawing of this distinction, with the poor of the 'underclass' viewed as inhabiting an alien and unapproachable world, different from everybody else, that marks one of the first steps in the new conception of poverty.

With the re-emergence of more individually determinist explanations of poverty has also disappeared any semblance of compassion or even charity. Even during the 1960s, when proponents of the 'culture of poverty' tried, somewhat unsuccessfully, to define poverty as the result of a distinctive sub-culture passed on from one generation to the next, there was a belief that this culture was at least in part the product of poverty itself, and that attempts could and should be made to break the cycle and reintegrate the poor back into the mainstream. The 'underclass' on the other hand are seen as a disease that is largely beyond cure. This constitutes the second feature in the changing conception of the poor whereby the most vulnerable and impoverished are condemned to studious neglect on the grounds that their plight is due primarily to the wilful attitudes or the inescapable biology of the individuals themselves: they can be dealt with only by punishment, control and containment. It is a line of thinking which echoes precisely with the Charity Organisation Society's (COS) distinction between the 'helpable and unhelpable' destitute developed in late Victorian Britain. Then, as now, it was argued that there were sections of the poor who were beyond help and to try to assist them through social welfare was simply throwing good money after bad. According to Bernard Bosanquet, the leading intellectual of the COS, the very idea that something could be done to improve the condition of the 'residuum' was

> in and by itself a potent factor in the creation of the miserable class whose existence we deplore; and all attempts to palliate the mischief by twining ropes of sand in pretending to organise the unorganisable material simply aggravates the disease by furnishing that partial and discontinuous employment which is the poison that corrupts these people's lives.
>
> (Bosanquet 1895: 113–14)

So it is at the end of the twentieth century that the myth of the 'dependency culture' has been used as a rationale for cutting spending on what one commentator has referred to as 'the murderous young underclass now being created by a large chunk of the incredibly growing £80 billion spent each year on misnamed "social security"' (Norman Macrae, *Sunday Times* 25 April 1993). Or as Bruce Anderson, adviser to successive Conservative prime ministers in the 1980s and 1990s, put it: 'We are in the grip of the post-modern vagabond. We have expensively constructed slums full of layabouts and sluts whose progeny are two-legged beasts. We cannot cure this by family, religion and self-help. So we will have to rely on repression' (Cited Davies 1997: 303).

The essentialism that sees poverty as the product of some innate anti-social characteristic further dictates that there is little to be understood about the poor or the reasons for their poverty. As the Conservative Home Secretary Kenneth Clarke put it, 'it is no good permanently finding excuses for a section of the population who are essentially nasty pieces of work' (*Independent* 28 February 1993). That explanations are seen as mere 'excuses', and that accumulated knowledge and research into poverty and its links with crime or social breakdown are dismissed out of hand and seen as having no relevance for the making of policy, constitutes a third feature of the new redefinition of poverty that has come to have immense ramifications for social policy and the structures of the British state.

## Reshaping social policy

During the last quarter of the twentieth century, social policy has taken on a more authoritarian, less compassionate and more coercive tone. This shift in policy has been more marked in some areas of policy than in others: just as the concept of the 'underclass' has been used to identify particular groups of the poor – single mothers, black people, the long-term unemployed or the young – so the coercive tilt in state policy has been directed at these groups in particular, and at the poorest of the poor, to configure what we might call, in place of the welfare state, the disciplinary state.

It is certainly true that since the rise to power of the new right within the Conservative party, and in its governments after 1979, few areas of the former welfare state have escaped untouched. The health service and the education system, while denied the resources necessary to meet the demands placed upon them, have been subject to the introduction of market forces, to 'cost efficiencies' and the increased exploitation of their workforces, and to greater centralisation and less democratic forms of control. But it is in those areas of state policy that deal predominantly with the poor – in social work, the means-tested benefit system and the criminal justice system – that some of the most profound changes have taken place.

The reasons for these changes, and the means of accomplishing them, are many and varied, and will form the focus of subsequent chapters. But what unites them is a view that state welfare itself has been a primary cause of the growth of an 'underclass' and its anti-social behaviour. Charles Murray puts this at the heart of his analysis:

> In the 1960s and 1970s social policy in Britain fundamentally changed what makes sense. The changes did not affect the mature as much as the young. They affected the affluent hardly at all. Rather, the rules of the game changed fundamentally for low-income young people. Behaviour changed along with the rules.
>
> (Murray 1990: 25)

Behind this lies a particular view of human nature – or at least of the nature of the poor – which sees them as essentially barbaric and undisciplined, requiring the firm hand of social sanction in order to maintain respect for the law, for the institutions of marriage or the family, or for the work ethic, and easily dissuaded from following these moral codes should the state appear to offer an alternative:

> Little boys don't naturally grow up to be responsible fathers and husbands. They don't naturally grow up knowing how to get up in the morning at the same time and go to work. They don't naturally grow up thinking that work is not just a way to make money . . . And little boys do not reach adolescence naturally wanting to refrain from sex, just as little girls don't become adolescents naturally wanting to refrain from having babies.
>
> (Murray 1990: 13)

As a result, so it is argued, changes in state social policy that took place during the 1960s and 1970s were corrupting of the morals of poor people. In particular the relative increase in the value of state benefits provided to lone parents meant that single parenthood 'went from being "extremely punishing" to "not so bad"' (Murray 1990: 30). This was a theme that was to be taken up by a succession of government ministers in the early 1990s, who saw in the growth of state welfare the reasons for the rise in single parenthood that has been a significant feature of British and other societies over the past decades. Thus according to Tom Sackville, then a junior health minister:

> The existence of a very comprehensive benefits and free housing system has reinforced the conclusion that anyone can have a baby at any time, regardless of their means and of the circumstances in which they can bring up their babies.
>
> (*Observer* 14 November 1993)

When Secretary of State for Wales, John Redwood similarly argued that there was a widespread belief amongst the young that 'the illegitimate child is the passport to a council flat and a benefit income' (*Independent* 14 August 1995), while the Secretary of State for Social Security, Peter Lilley, delighted the baying audience at successive Conservative Party conferences with his equally fatuous remarks about young unmarried mothers. The Home Secretary Michael Howard went further, blaming single mothers for the fact that 'children, instead of learning the difference between right and wrong, instead concentrate on how not to get caught' (*Independent* 20 November 1993). Equally, New Labour's Home Secretary Jack Straw argued in 1998:

There is not much doubt in the minds of a lot of us that a combination of the collapse of unskilled and semi-skilled employment, the availability of housing for single people from the age of sixteen, and the benefit system have created an environment in which the natural checks that existed before on teenagers becoming pregnant and having children, and keeping them, have gone in some areas. We have got to rebalance that.

(*Observer* 1 February 1998)

In such ways the image of an 'underclass', locked into dependency on the state and growing in numbers, is constructed and used as a basis for policy changes. Characteristically, these changes affect many more than just those singled out for criticism. The vagueness and imprecision of the concept of the underclass makes it very elastic: what in this case began as an attack on teenage unmarried mothers was extended to a much wider range of people. In 1996 the government's promise to begin to tackle 'the problem' of teenage unmarried motherhood took shape with the 1996 Housing Act: characteristically this ended the automatic entitlement not only of young unmarried mothers, but of all other priority homeless groups to permanent public housing.

The idea that the 1960s brought about a profound cultural revolution in attitudes towards the family, work and respect for authority and the law – the results of which Britain is seen as reaping in the moral decay of the 1990s – is another theme to which we will return. But for a number of commentators, not only on the far right, the effects were most damning for the poor. Thus for the Labour MP Frank Field, long-standing chair of the House of Commons Select Committee on Social Security, the change in moral codes that was seen as a product of the 'permissive' 1960s is also seen as a decisive turning point in affecting the behaviour of the poor:

All too many of today's political leaders were active supporters of a relativist code of conduct which refused to rank human behaviour. It is safer to preach and act such a line of course if daddy has a big bank balance to fall back upon. But at a time when the financial advantages of marriage have lessened, when jobs paying family wages are on the decline, priorities about childrearing have come under attack. This left the poorest and least able bearing the full brunt of this particular vicious era of political correctness, that single parenthood is equal, if not superior, to two-parent families as a unit in which to raise children.

(Field 1996: 113)

Central to this explanation is the view that the poor respond to these changes in ways that others do not: 'Such benefits don't have much effect on affluent women – the benefit rate is far below what they consider their needs . . . for poor women, however, the benefit level can be quite salient in deciding whether having a baby is feasible' (Murray 1990: 29). In the same way, 'those with brawn and little developed intelligence' (Field 1996: 17) are considered to be particularly susceptible to the corrupting influence of state benefits. This is seen as particularly so for the young unemployed, whose rejection of the work ethic and preference for a life on state benefits mean that even a return to 'full employment' will not solve the problem. According to Field:

> We've got a number of young people who are now outside the labour market, who've created their own world, partly though crime, partly through drugs, partly through drawing welfare, and who are not prepared to join Great Britain Ltd again on the terms that we offer.
> (BBC Radio 4 Analysis 3 December 1992)

He was to be appointed by Tony Blair as Minister for Welfare Reform in the New Labour government of 1997 to 'think the unthinkable'.

For Field, whose Christian fundamentalism allies him to the dominant religiously-influenced group within the Labour government, human beings are fallible – 'we are less than perfect creatures' (Field 1996: 112) – and the temptations of benefits, and their ability to corrupt human behaviour, are many. Unlike the view held by the far right, this view – like that of a number of Field's New Labour colleagues – is not that all state provision is corrupting, but rather that certain forms are, while others may legitimately play a useful role. 'Welfare', he argued, 'should openly reward good behaviour and it should be used to enhance those roles which the country values' (Field 1996: 9).

Yet the analysis of the problem remains essentially similar. It is the growth of those means-tested benefits on which the poor have to rely that has had the greatest corrupting influence: 'Means tests are the cancer within the welfare state, rotting decent values and overwhelming the honesty and dignity of recipients in almost equal proportions' (Field 1996: 9). Arguing that they are 'steadily recruiting a nation of cheats and liars' (Field 1996: 11) means-tested benefits are thus seen as contributing to the formation of the dependency culture and the growth of an 'underclass':

> By undermining the character of the poor, means tests create a fertile ground for the 'yob culture', which is one of the underclass's

distinguishing marks for many male members, and for some females as well. Crime and drugs, themselves often linked together, need to be added. Indeed the underclass, at its strongest point, is fed by unemployment, the abuse of welfare, crime and drugs.

(Field 1996: 18)

The absence of compassion in these new discourses on poverty and the so-called underclass cannot be allowed to pass without comment. It says much about the confidence of political elites that they feel so unrestrained in their moral condemnation of those who already suffer most from the poverty and inequality that late twentieth-century capitalism has created. We now live in a society in which it is not regarded as unthinkable for political leaders to say virtually what they like about those whose daily lives are circumscribed by struggle and hardship, compounded by institutionalised and routinised abuse. As Nick Davies observed:

Every time a government minister from any party stands up and declares war on the welfare state, every time some respected thinker jeers at the idea of equality or contrives a case for stripping the poor of yet more benefits, they give a cloak of respectability to this hardness.

(Davies 1997: 300)

For those on the receiving end of such insults the pain is often palpable, as John Pilger illustrated during his discussion with Amy and Trisha, two single mothers living a 'no frills' life on welfare:

'. . . Scroungers', said Amy. 'It's a hateful thing to call us, and it's not true. They don't *know* how hard we try to get jobs; they don't know that you're turned down the moment they know you've been in care. They don't know how few jobs there are, and what a con a lot of them are' . . . Amy seems close to tears.

(Pilger 1998: 103)

Of course they don't know. For these elites, well removed from the consequences of their actions, the new discourse on the poor and poverty self-evidently rules out any need to enter into dialogue with those who are abused. Given their construction as worthless and as counting for nothing they are seen as having little of any value to say about their condition. The so-called debates about poverty, or 'the underclass', or welfare dependency, whether in parliament or in the media, are consistently characterised by the absence of the poor themselves. Their voices, stories and perspectives scarcely feature. They appear only as objects.

## Capitalism and poverty

The depiction of the poorest as a degenerate and incorrigible 'underclass' can only be understood in the context of increasing inequality and levels of poverty at the end of the twentieth century. During the 1980s the number of people defined – in conventional terms – as in poverty in Britain increased four-fold. By the mid-1990s over one in four of the population (including one in three children) lived on or below half of average national income. The growing inequality between rich and poor in Britain during this period was greater than in any other developed country, and the speed of its polarisation matched only by New Zealand. As for the USA, the world's richest country, the gap between rich and poor remains the greatest (Brenner 1998: 211).

Such statistics, however, understate the real extent of the change that has taken place, and obscure its wider political significance. Growing poverty and inequality have afflicted the lives of many millions more than just those conventionally defined as in poverty. On such definitions, the poor are isolated as a minority, their poverty defined by an arbitrary and often extremely meagre level of income. In the USA this poverty line, determined by estimates of minimum nutritional standards, falls far below what people actually need to live on. In Britain, no such 'official' definition of poverty has ever existed, although the measures traditionally used are similarly mean and unrealistic. While, even on these definitions, the number of poor has grown dramatically, the effects of poverty and of the dynamics that create it – the growth of insecurity and declining incomes from work, the reductions in state benefits, and the transfer of resources through changes in taxation and other measures to benefit the rich – have resulted in a deterioration in the lives, relative living standards and working conditions of most people. It is in the management of the consequences of this that the labelling of the poorest as an 'underclass', and their treatment as less than deserving of sympathy and respect, has its true significance.

For almost exactly a century both academic and, more lately, popular understandings of poverty have seen it as defined by a particular level of income. Before then it had been most widely understood, not as any particular level of income, but as a relationship of social class. Thus the nineteenth-century social reformer Nassau Senior spoke of

the unfortunate double meaning of the word *poor* . . . In its widest acceptation it is opposed to the word *rich*; and in its most common use it includes all, except the higher and middle classes –

in short, all who derive their subsistence solely from manual labour.

(Senior 1865: 67)

Poverty is a relative concept: it cannot be understood in isolation, as a fact that exists independently of comparison with others. On the contrary, poverty only makes sense in comparison with wealth, in the same way that short only makes sense in comparison with tall. They are both different sides of the same coin, but the relationship between poverty and wealth goes further than this. One is not merely a static mirror-image of the other. Rather they are bound up in a dynamic relationship in which one produces the other. Another early nineteenth-century political economist, Patrick Colquhoun, who amongst others was attempting to understand and theorise for the first time the workings of an emerging industrial capitalism, summed up this relationship precisely:

> Poverty is that state and condition in society where the individual has no surplus labour in store, and, consequently, no property but what is derived from the constant exercise of industry in the various occupations of life; or in other words, it is the state of every one who must labour for subsistence.
>
> Poverty is therefore a most necessary and indispensable ingredient in society, without which nations and communities could not exist in a state of civilisation. It is the lot of man – it is the source of wealth, since without poverty there would be no labour, and without labour there could be no riches, no refinement, no comfort, and no benefit to those who may be possessed of wealth.
>
> (cited Rose 1971: 47)

In this sense poverty is, in the scale of human history, a modern phenomenon, originating in the division of society – brought about in Britain from the Middle Ages onwards, although in most parts of the world of much more recent origin – between owners of wealth on the one hand and a propertyless working class, compelled by its lack of property to seek employment and to produce and increase this wealth on the other. Although earlier forms of society, of feudalism or slavery for example, contained their own forms of inequality, the modern condition of poverty emerges only with the development of capitalism.

The private ownership of wealth that characterises capitalist production, the ownership of the land, factories, machinery, offices and shops on which the majority depend for their employment thus frames the condition of poverty, and together these two seemingly natural, but in reality historically specific, features provide the dynamic through which capitalism has developed.

Most statistics on the distribution of wealth are based on property which can be sold on the market, and may include not only stocks and shares, the ownership of factories and other means of production through which wealth and income are created, but also people's houses and other saleable assets, even though the latter constitute a very different form of wealth. But although these statistics are thus limited and in other ways incomplete – for the rich have good cause, and much opportunity, to obscure their holdings of wealth – the evidence they present is incontrovertible. In Britain at the end of the twentieth century the richest 10 per cent of the population own 65 per cent of marketable wealth, excluding dwellings, while half the population between them have only 6 per cent (Office of National Statistics 1995). In the USA the distribution is even more extreme: a mere 1 per cent of the population owning 42 per cent of private wealth. If distributed equally, each American household would have wealth to the value of $220,000; yet for the 'average' American household, that at the mid-point of the distribution of the population, median wealth in 1991 amounted to $36,000 (the share of the majority constituted mostly by the value of their houses), while for the 'average' African-American household it was a mere $4,000 (US Bureau of Census 1994).

The ownership of wealth, and with it the power to dictate the economic fortunes of everyone else, has remained in the hands of a minority throughout capitalism's history. Changes in its distribution have largely been confined to shifts within this minority: from the richest one to the next 5 or 10 per cent, and only to a much more limited extent has it extended any further during the course of the twentieth century. Yet even this limited progress towards the myth of a 'property-owning democracy' has in the last quarter of the twentieth century been reversed, as the rich have become richer, and the very rich richest of all. Between 1979 and 1992, 99 per cent of all new wealth created in the USA was claimed by only one-fifth of the population (boosting the share of total wealth owned by the richest 1 per cent from 23 per cent to 42 per cent), while the remaining 1 per cent of new wealth was left to be distributed amongst the remaining 80 per cent of the population (Wolff 1995). The much-proclaimed 'trickle-down' effect, used as a justification by both Reagan and Thatcher governments for the further enrichment of the wealthy minority on the grounds that the majority, and even the poorest, would ultimately benefit, predictably failed to materialise.

While wealth begets more wealth, so it also affects income. It is not only that the rich receive income simply from owning wealth. It is also that those without wealth – and the majority of the population in all capitalist societies own no appreciable wealth – are as a result required to earn an income in order to survive. It is this relationship to wealth and the means of producing it, and the constant economic insecurity it threatens, which is important. In this respect it matters little whether a society's wealth is owned by individuals, or corporations, controlled by investment fund managers or even by the state. Although important in other respects, this does not change this fundamental relationship of capitalism and the necessity it creates for people to work to earn an income.

Some, like the 'middle' classes who stand between the owners of wealth and the working classes, do this comfortably, although even then most have no more margin than the equivalent of a few months' salary to keep them from penury should some catastrophe befall them. Others work constantly to keep their heads above water, spurred by rising standards of living and consumerism in 'a perpetual never-satisfied desire for something better than anything that is ever realised' (Rea 1912: 10). Many, and now in increasing numbers, fail even to achieve this, and are spurred by the threat of poverty into work that does not even provide for the basic necessities of life – or, unable to work or to find it, are left dependent on the mercies of a state benefit system that increasingly strives to shake off any responsibility. It is this fundamental characteristic of modern poverty, of 'poverty amidst plenty' that serves ultimately as the motor of the capitalist labour market and its incentives to work. It is this also that makes poverty, and the continuing threat of poverty, a necessary and inescapable feature of capitalist society. 'Those that get their living by their daily labour', argued Bernard deMandeville in 1728, 'have nothing to stir them up to be serviceable but their wants which it is prudence to relieve but folly to cure' (cited Marx 1974: 576).

Political necessity has made the relief – although never the abolition – of this condition a feature of most advanced capitalist societies. The reality of a market economy – which in Britain produces an average income for the poorest fifth of the population of less than £2,000 per household per year (Office of National Statistics 1995), and for some no income at all – has resulted in the creation of an elaborate system of state transfer of resources through various forms of taxation, social security and assistance schemes. For the most part these transfers have been designed to take less from the rich than from the rest: to transfer income from the poor to the poorest, the young to the old, the healthy to the sick, and the employed to the unemployed. Above all they have been designed, while relieving to an extent the threat of destitution for most (although as we shall see, by no means all) of the poor, not to interfere with the fundamental incentives that poverty creates.

The radical restructuring of taxation and social-security spending engineered by both the Thatcher and Reagan governments and their successors since 1979, coupled with an offensive by employers to restrain wages and undermine working conditions, have exacerbated this effect, squeezing yet further the poor and those on middle incomes, and intensifying conflicts between them. As a result an increasing proportion of the population have seen their relative position decline. The poorest, as we shall see, have suffered the most, but in both countries the fall in relative incomes – relative to the growing wealth and incomes of the rich – affected a substantial majority. Not only do they have an even smaller share of wealth, they have faced declining living standards: by the mid-1990s two-thirds of the British population depended on an income lower than the national average.

It is in this context that poverty has to be understood and the differential treatment of the poor explained. Poverty is not an isolated event, periodically and mysteriously befalling a minority of the population. It is rather a condition of economic life which produces a continuum of standards of living. Its pressures are felt most keenly by the poorest, but are not limited to those who fall below an arbitrary and minimal level of income. The pressures of modern poverty are never entirely removed from the majority of people, and although they struggle, with greater or lesser success, to keep their heads above water – some of them comfortably so – the threat of redundancy, or of an incapacitating illness, threatens to reveal in full and devastating force the fundamental economic insecurity, the chasm of poverty, that capitalism has created for all but the rich.

It is also in this context that the treatment of the poorest impacts on the rest. The higher up the continuum of poverty people are, the less they may feel the immediate chill of its icy draught, but they are never immune. Increased competition for work, and its consequent lowering of wages at the bottom of the labour market, filters upwards; the reduction or withdrawal of benefits for those at the bottom increases the insecurity and pressure not only directly on them, but on all those who fear to slip down the continuum. As Nancy Hollander has written of the USA, although her remarks apply equally well to Britain:

> For the first time in the country's history the next generation will have less opportunity and a lower standard of living and will experience more social violence than their parents. Although people in every part of the country exert great effort to make meaning out of

their work, to build loving bonds among family and friends, and to strengthen their community ties, the hurdles to these aspirations loom larger all the time. More people live in fear of losing their jobs, of not being able to pay for their children's education, of not being able to care for their ageing parents, and of losing everything they have spent a lifetime creating. The vast majority who experience these fears are individuals and families who keep doggedly on track, although the road is getting tougher. Their work ethic and family values are threatened not by their personal moral deterioration, but by a system that is wiping out decent jobs, driving down wages, and eliminating social policies that once supported rather than sabotaged the American family.

(Hollander 1997: 224)

It is a testament to the powerful stigmatisation of poverty, which in Britain has been a consistent consequence of state policy for the past 600 years, as well as to the success during the last 100 years in redefining poverty, not as the necessary condition of a class, but as the misfortune – wilful or otherwise – of a minority, that most people do not see themselves as poor, although most would gain from an equalisation of incomes. On the contrary, the effects of the stigmatisation of poverty have been to lead people to seek to distance themselves from those beneath them. The drawing of a poverty line arbitrarily cuts off those who supposedly are poor from those who seemingly are not, even though the circumstances of those immediately above the line are little if any different from those below. The holding of the minority of poor as responsible through lack of effort, or intelligence, for their own poverty serves to justify the efforts and sacrifices that others make to keep above them. Thus the poor as a whole are fragmented and divided: each layer striving to keep afloat, justifying their success in doing so as the result of their own effort and initiative, and seeing the failure of others as the justifiable consequence of their lack of effort. Rarely, although for good reason, does anyone look sufficiently far upwards to the worlds of the rich, and still less to the mechanisms and processes through which this order is maintained.

It is tempting for the married couple who struggle to earn a living, to pay the rent or mortgage, to keep up with the growing burden of taxation, to keep their children out of trouble, and to save for their old age, and who succeed in doing so (if they succeed at all) only through immense personal cost and sacrifice, through long hours of work, little relaxation, and few enjoyments in life, to see 'the single mother on welfare' or the non-working household dependent on benefits not only as morally less responsible than themselves, but also as somehow contributing to the severity of the struggle and the sacrifices that they themselves have to make. The temptation is greatly reinforced in the media and by politicians who daily blame the so-called 'dependency culture' and the cost of welfare spending for the increased burden of taxation, who decry 'scroungers' and the 'work-shy', and who make the least powerful objects of derision and scorn. It is certainly easier than to look in the other direction: to the little-publicised activities of a small minority – a minority whose power and wealth is anyway apparently as 'natural', inevitable and unassailable as it is great.

It is on this powerful dynamic that concepts such as 'the underclass' play most effectively. As the living standards of the majority have fallen in relative terms, and for the poorest actually gone backwards, the view that the poorest and most impoverished are themselves responsible – that they constitute indeed a different and alien species from the rest of the hard-working, sober, thrifty and law-abiding population – both justifies their neglect and acts powerfully to encourage the hard-working to distance themselves yet further from such a fate. The labelling and treatment of the poorest as an 'underclass' thus acts both as an example and a threat. It is a dynamic which in its various guises has attempted to keep the poorest isolated, the poor from realising that they have interests in common, and the rich from being confronted, for the most part even identified, as the beneficiaries of the process.

The victims of poverty are not confined to that 20 or 30 per cent of the population who fall below the poverty line. Even by such a measure, the fluctuation in living standards over an individual's lifetime means that many more people will, at least at some stage in their lives, find themselves struggling to make ends meet. But this struggle does not end once people have risen above this threshold. For many, staying above the threshold is a feat that is achieved only at immense personal cost. Long hours of work, the growing necessity in many families for both partners to take a job and the growing number of people having to work at two or more jobs leave little time, or energy, for the enjoyment of life, for time to spend with children, partners or friends.

The changing nature of work itself is also part of the problem. Growth in the extremes of poverty, and in particular the growth – and maintenance – of high levels of unemployment are mirrored in a deterioration in not only the wages but also the conditions and relationships of many of those in work. During the 1980s and 1990s job insecurity has become a spectre hanging over the heads of millions employed in all sectors and at most levels of the British economy. Employers have not been slow to take advantage of this situation. The rights of those at work, especially trade-union rights, have been either removed or eroded as the 'right to manage' has imposed new forms of discipline, increased the speed and tempo of work, and exacted a greater toll from the work-force. Summary dismissal, casualisation and the threat of redundancy have created in many workplaces a climate of insecurity and fear. Added to this has been a widespread deskilling of labour as workers have lost control over what they do, and as new routinised forms of service employment have replaced older, no less arduous, but often more meaningful forms of work.

The stress – both physical and mental – that this has imposed on a great part of the population is incalculable. But the evidence of it is everywhere: in road rage, the evident fractiousness between parents and children, the retreat into individualised routes of escape, whether through drugs (legal and illegal), addiction to the soporific effects of television or the equally desperate dream of winning the lottery, and in mounting levels of sickness, absenteeism and suicide.

But the reality is that for the overwhelming majority there is no escape. The pressures and threat of poverty inexorably drive people back the next day to the same monotony, humiliation and degradation of the human spirit that has come to characterise work in contemporary capitalism. These experiences are of course greatest for the lowest paid, but we cannot seriously suggest that they affect only those who live below the poverty line.

## Poverty as a social relation

To see poverty as a social relation is to see it as much more than just a level of income. Although in the final analysis poverty is about resources – and the power to command resources – this does not restrict us to issues of economics. Human relations are at one and the same time economic, social, political, cultural and psychological. The fragmentation of human experience into different disciplinary categories may be intellectually convenient, but remains an artificial imposition on and division of social life, and may often serve to obscure important similarities and interconnections. Although the study of poverty may now be largely framed within what we have come to term economic relationships, economic relations are themselves both social and political. They are – despite the apparent neutrality of the market – relations between people, and embody relationships of power, of superiority and inferiority, security and insecurity. The nature of these relations is as crucial in determining the experience of poverty as is any particular level of income.

In general to be poor is to be confronted by a society which condemns you as a failure. Based on such a perception, state policy towards the poor has been generally hostile. Optimists may point to the periodic bouts of social reform that have punctuated this history, the surfacing of more sympathetic attitudes and policies, at least towards some of the poor, that have restored some dignity and understanding. But in the time-span of poverty and given the scale of the problem we have to face the fact that such developments have been often temporary, short-lived and of little effect. Poverty has not gone away; rather it is increasing. Punitive attitudes once again drive the policy agenda, and the denigration of the poor continues.

The parsimoniousness and pettiness of the benefit system is a constant in the lives of many of the poor. When, as in the experience of the Social Fund, it refuses help to people because they are too poor to pay back what little they are offered it reveals a callousness that is more than just accidental or the result of some unfortunate administrative error. The belittling and degradation of claimants is a systematic feature of the way the state treats those most dependent upon it, and as the conditions of the labour market have deteriorated for the working poor, so have the conditions for those on benefit. The indifference shown to the consequences of this for both groups spells only one thing: that the poor do not count.

We are well to be indignant, better to be outraged, but we should not be surprised at this. Capitalism, while it creates and feeds on poverty, is also challenged by it. If capitalism is to avoid the challenge, poverty must be managed and contained, and the greater the amount and severity of poverty, the greater the need to explain it away, to put the blame on the poor themselves as an incorrigible 'underclass', and to punish them accordingly.

While some may avoid, and even actively resist, the labels placed upon them, few can avoid the more bodily damage that poverty inflicts. Here again, it is not merely level of income that counts. As Richard Wilkinson's research (1996) convincingly shows, it is the relationships between poverty and wealth, and the degree of inequality within a particular society, that are the major determinants not only of physical but also of mental health. Poverty is a corrosive which acts not only through the effects of malnutrition and unhealthy living and working conditions, but also through those social relationships which depict the poor as worthless.

Surviving poverty is thus not only a matter of trying to balance an inadequate budget. It is also having to deal with the social and psychological stress, with insecurity, social isolation and the often thinly disguised contempt of the more powerful. In a paper presented to the Copenhagen Summit on Social Development, Robert Chambers reported several pieces of research into third-world poverty that aimed to discover the priorities and definitions of the poor themselves. Amongst these, research by Tony Beck in West Bengal revealed that respondents 'did not hesitate in saying that for them respect was more important than food, and that "without respect food won't go into the stomach"' (cited Chambers 1994). Elsewhere, researchers found that even where the poor were worse off in economic terms than they had been ten or fifteen years earlier, by their own definitions they were better off: 'more income' ranking only ninth or tenth in a list of priorities headed by other concerns such as 'more time at home' and relationships with neighbours. As Chambers remarks, 'humiliation and self-respect do not lend themselves to measurement, are in practice not measured, and so, for normal professionals, barely exist and rarely count' (ibid.).

It would be ridiculous to deny the importance of income to the poor, whether in the third world or in the so-called developed world. It is, after all, the difference in income and wealth that makes the aged, unemployed or single-parent status of half the British royal family qualitatively different from that of their poorer counterparts. But income is not the only determinant of poverty, nor is it the only or necessarily the most oppressive feature in the experience of the poor. Poverty may be created by an economic system whose inequalities in the ownership of wealth and in the distribution of income are self-perpetuating, but it is maintained by a set of social relationships that keep this system in place.

## The truth about 'the underclass'

The vilification and demonisation of an 'underclass', as John Macnicol has argued, reveals more about the fears and preoccupations of those responsible for it than it does the truth about the poor themselves. These fears – about the declining respect for authority, the disintegration of the patriarchal nuclear family, the advances made by women and black people, the erosion of the work ethic – are in part a response to contemporary social change: changes which are by no means confined to the poor, although it is on the poor that the burden of blame for them is laid. Underlying all these is also a common fear, as old as capitalism itself, that the attachment of the working population to the virtues and disciplines demanded by capitalist society are at best tenuous, and constantly in need of reinforcement.

Throughout its history, the defenders of capitalism have feared that this discipline is easily undermined, and have seen the institutions of work, marriage and the family as central to its maintenance. With this has gone the fear that those who – by choice or fate – fall outside its regulatory mechanisms cannot be controlled. As Raymond Plant recalls:

> The issue, however, is not a new one. The spectre of an underclass has haunted critics and defenders of capitalism for nearly two centuries. Of course, pre-capitalist societies knew abject poverty and destitution, but there are features of industrial capitalism that transform sections of the poor into an underclass, in the sense that they not only lack resources, but are alienated from society. This puts them beyond social control.
>
> (*Times* 15 May 1990)

In similar vein, Thomas Mackay, a leading authority on Poor Law reform at the beginning of the twentieth century, discussed the problem of the 'residuum':

> It is not a question of those who fall, but rather of those who never rise, who, though they have periods of prosperity, use their advantage for making their hand-to-mouth life for the moment more profuse, and who have no conception of any other sort of life. They decline altogether to submit themselves to the teaching of the economic order. The economically disciplined class fear poverty, and, taking some pains to avoid it, as a rule succeed in avoiding its severest forms. The main difficulty of the situation arises from the fact that for the undisciplined poverty has no terrors.
>
> (Mackay 1902: 285)

It is the fear that such 'resolutely proletarian attitudes' (ibid.) will extend to and undermine the fragile attachment of the remainder – that 'the restraining influence will break down much more rapidly for the knowledge that Smith's children are better cared for since he gave up the battle, and so the mischief spreads down the street like an epidemic' (Bosanquet 1896: 73) – that constitutes the 'underclass' as a cancer to be eradicated.

The construction of an image of 'the underclass' both as different from the rest of the population and as responsible for a decline in moral order, for increasing crime, the disintegration of family relationships and growing poverty is a distortion of reality that would merit centre place in George Orwell's *Nineteen Eighty-four*. It is a construction that

is all the more audacious, more cruel and at the same time more compelling to the extent to which it has taken the victims of poverty and
turned them into villains. The concept of the 'underclass' fundamentally misrepresents what is happening in society, blaming the poor for
much more complex and wide-ranging social changes and problems,
and in pinpointing the victims of these processes caricatures and abuses
them as an example to others.

Certainly the last quarter of the twentieth century has been a period
of significant social change. The return of mass unemployment, the
casualisation and increased insecurity of work, the destruction of families and communities through economic decline, dislocation and stress
form the main focus of this book. But there have also been major
changes in culture and in family life: the ideal of life-long monoga-
mous marriage has long ceased to be the norm. People now marry later
in life, if at all, and are more likely to separate or divorce, often to form
other family relationships. Greater variety in family and household
forms, and less permanency in their arrangements, characterise most
developed countries. In Britain one-third of all children are now born
outside of marriage, a proportion that continues to rise; half of all
marriages now end in divorce, and more couples live together without
marrying, both heterosexual and homosexual, while an increasing
number of households consist of single people or multiple occupancy.
These are significant and widespread changes, the product of a complex
range of factors. To identify the growth of single mothers as the cause
of these changes reveals a profound ignorance of social phenomena.

Single parenthood, as the British royal family amply demonstrates, is
not of course confined to the very poor. Here, as with other elements of
its description, the concept of the 'underclass' reveals its profound class
bias. The ideal form of the bourgeois nuclear family has never attained
universal acceptance, especially amongst the British aristocracy: its
record of extra-marital affairs, of infidelity and sexual licentiousness
would be enough to fill volumes. Equally the growth of sexual experi-
mentation, the lessening of social taboos against gay and lesbian
relationships, the growing independence of women and their increasing
right to choose whether or when to marry and have children, and the
weakening power of patriarchy, have extended across all social classes.
If anything, a range of surveys and other research shows the poorest to
be more conformist, more attached to the values of 'family life' than the
bulk of the population (Heath 1992). Yet it is on the poorest alone that
proponents of an 'underclass' have concentrated.

The same is true of crime, whose growth has been focused on the
poor at a time when the crimes of the rich and powerful have flourished

for the most part unchallenged. Revelations of misconduct, fraud and theft within the major financial institutions of the City of London indicate a cost to the British economy that far outweighs the petty thefts of the poor, while, like the law itself, the social violence of factory closures or the damage done by currency speculators often does not merit a mention in the mainstream media. So too it is with unemployment. The idle rich rarely figure alongside discussions of the idle poor, yet it is only amongst the former that unemployment is a matter of choice. For the poor, unemployment is a catastrophe, and its growth the result of structural changes in the economy that have significantly reduced the opportunities in particular for unskilled work. Once again, surveys demonstrate that the so-called 'underclass' has a fierce attachment to the work ethic, if for no other reason than economic necessity (Gaillie 1994; MacDonald 1994; Payne and Payne 1994). If there is a revulsion against work, this is hardly surprising. For most people, work in the 1980s and 1990s has become even more pressured, exhausting and less satisfying; but the option voluntarily to give up work, to take early retirement and to move to the sun remains overwhelmingly the prerogative of those who can afford to do so.

At the same time proponents of 'the underclass' ignore the effects of the dismantling of the welfare state in exacerbating the problems for which the existence of welfare is held to blame. The pauperisation of the poor owes as much to changes in state policy as it does to the restructuring of the economy. Cuts in benefit leave many with no alternative other than to turn to crime. When in 1987 the Conservative election manifesto promised that it would take steps 'to ensure that those under eighteen who deliberately choose to remain unemployed are not eligible for benefit' (cited Andrews and Jacobs 1990: 79) it created a situation of increasing desperation. Since then 16- and 17-year-olds unable to find a job or a place on a training scheme, without families or with families unable or unwilling to support them, have formed a growing number of the destitute and homeless. In 1994, 97,000 such young people had no job and no training place, and only a quarter received any income, mostly in the form of the tightly controlled Severe Hardship Allowance payable only to those at serious risk of abuse or of significant harm to health (Unemployment Unit 1994). Many inevitably found themselves on the streets, forced to turn to begging, theft and more damaging forms of exploitation in order to survive:

Home Office figures show that between 1989 and 1993 nearly 1,500 young people under 18 were convicted of offences relating to prostitution and a further 1,800 were cautioned. The numbers are rising . . . According to the Chief Executive of the Church of England charity the Children's Society, 'prostitution is very often a survival strategy for young people on the streets who have no money, food or shelter'.

(*Guardian* 18 October 1995)

Similarly the attempt to restore a more restrictive sexual morality, to reverse what was seen as the legacy of 'permissiveness' of the 1960s, has itself compounded the issue of illegitimacy. Whether the rise in illegitimacy is a problem, or whether it represents a welcome weakening of the restrictive institutions of marriage and patriarchy, is a matter of political opinion. Whether people have a choice in the matter is, however, also a matter of education and knowledge. The introduction of restrictions on sexual education in schools, on the provision of birth control and on abortion have all reduced the opportunities available especially to young people to make informed choices. To the extent that there is a problem in the rise of births outside wedlock, especially to teenage girls, it is these factors that are significant rather than the supposed amoral values of an 'underclass' (Selman and Glendenning 1994/5).

Housing policy too has served to concentrate the poorest in some of the worst housing conditions, pushing beyond the limit the ability of many estates to cope with the accumulated consequences of poverty and social stress. The 'right to buy' introduced in the 1980s for public-sector housing was exercised most by the more mobile and affluent, leaving behind estates populated by the unemployed, the elderly and the relatively young. As one research report argued, 'this is leading to an ever-narrowing social base. Those with the lowest income, the worst social health and drug problems, are being concentrated in the social housing sector' (cited *Guardian* 13 February 1997). The *Guardian* editorial went on to point out:

Three decades ago the typical council housing estate still comprised a wide social mix. No longer. The right-to-buy policy . . . has combined with deep cuts to the housing programme to produce social housing estates more familiar to American than British policy-makers. The cycle is becoming self-perpetuating, with newcomers more disadvantaged than existing tenants . . . Three quarters of tenants moving in are aged between 16 and 29 . . . An increasing number of estates are not just difficult to manage and to let, but extremely difficult to live in.

(*Guardian* 13 February 1997)

To see the deterioration of such estates as the consequence of 'contamination' by the anti-social values of an 'underclass' is simply to pander to a reactionary politics and to ignore the deep-rooted nature of the problems that many poor communities have to live and cope with. The introduction of legislation such as that to evict 'anti-social' tenants, introduced on the same day this report was published, merely displaces the problem elsewhere.

Although the concept of an 'underclass' is nebulous and empirically unproven, it nevertheless has come to have significant political purchase. One reason for this has been its ability to take as examples those whose lives have been most disfigured and distorted by poverty and to generalise these into the characteristics of a whole population. If there is one partial truth on which the power of the new construction of poverty rests, it is that poverty can be wholly corrosive of human relationships, dignity and self-respect. That this is not the case for the vast majority of the poor is testament to the strength and determination of people to resist its brutalising effects, and to the culture of mutual support that has always characterised poverty. But a few are also defeated: the battle to maintain human dignity in the face of prolonged poverty, hopelessness and rejection is lost, and relationships with families, friends and neighbours are pushed beyond breaking point. It is hardly surprising that the social violence inflicted on poor people rebounds: that desperation, frustration and anger boil out in riots and rampage, or in apparently 'mindless' attacks on those in authority. The greater surprise is that this does not happen more often. More often the violence is turned further inwards, into deep depression, suicide or an ultimately self-destructive drug addiction which offers a short but fatal escape. To make those who are overwhelmed by the brutality of poverty an example of and to others constitutes the greatest abuse of the poor.

## Common sense

Whether the 'underclass' is defined in terms of attitudes to work and benefits, the spatial concentration of long-term unemployment, crime or single parenthood, what research is available simply does not support the notion that such a class exists. This pursuit of an ideological agenda in the face of limited, and even contradictory, evidence is, however, not new. During the inter-war depression, similar attempts to construct an image of the dangerous and degenerate poor were equally based upon impressionistic accounts in the absence of any hard evidence. As the Wood Report on Mental Deficiency noted, 'anyone who has extensive practical experience of social service would readily admit' that it exists, but 'we have comparatively little reliable data relating to the mental endowments and characteristics of this "social problem group"' (cited Macnicol 1987: 302). In similar vein, more contemporary commentators such as Melanie Phillips have argued that 'just because research doesn't identify an underclass in Britain doesn't mean it isn't there. It might just mean that academics haven't yet woken up to reality', while 'the professionals who work on the frontiers of disadvantage, by contrast, see it daily' (BBC Radio 4 Analysis 3 December 1992).

This pitting of the 'common sense' of those, unspecified, individuals who 'know' an 'underclass' exists against what is dismissed as the arcane world of academic research has become an increasingly worrying feature not only of the supposed existence of an 'underclass', but also of the formation of state policy itself. We shall take up this theme in subsequent chapters, to explore the ways in which the refashioning of social policy has involved a philistine repudiation of research and intellectual knowledge, and an attempt to silence and tame intellectuals and welfare professionals, held responsible, as in the *Sunday Times* editorial cited at the beginning of this chapter, for the supposed collapse of morality amongst the working-class poor. Here we simply note its consequences for the understanding and politics of poverty. The construction of 'the underclass' requires a silencing of those who contradict its individualising and victim-blaming approach. In place of the need for an understanding of the complex dynamics through which poverty is created and reproduced, and of its effects on individuals, families and communities, it offers simplistic nostrums that appeal to tabloid headlines and exacerbate the tensions and divisions that exist amongst the poor as a whole.

In many ways this has always been the case. The present politics of poverty reflect a fundamental continuity in the management and containment of the fundamental inequality of capitalism. Yet the present is also different from the past. Events at the end of the twentieth century have much in common with the 1920s and 1930s, the end of the nineteenth century, or the 1820s and 1830s: mass unemployment and growing poverty on the one hand, and an increasingly punitive reaction to its victims on the other. But the current reaction is taking place in a very different context. The establishment of a welfare state after 1945, for all its many limitations and shortcomings, changed the political map of countries like Britain. The post-war settlement between capital and labour introduced an unprecedented, if incomplete, level of security for ordinary people. It opened up avenues for education, for an increasing standard of living, and for attempts both to understand and to eradicate a wide range of social problems. That it largely failed to do so does not erase the possibilities it offered.

It was also for these reasons that the welfare state could not be sustained. It was less the economic costs of welfare – in Britain substantially lower than in many other and more successful capitalist economies – than its political consequences that were seen to be the problem. The increased confidence of ordinary people and their growing expectations, their demand to be treated decently as human beings, to be accorded rights and a fair share of the income and wealth they produced: these were not in themselves revolutionary, but they pushed the post-war settlement further than an increasingly global capitalism would allow. Those gains have now been taken back with a vengeance. There is probably no parallel in the history of British society when so much has been taken back and turned on its head in such a short time. Trade unions have been decimated and workers told to accept the dictates of management or else face the consequences. The welfare state has been demonised as a corrupting influence and 'welfare dependency' has entered political discourse as an evil to be eradicated. The language of welfare has been reinvented: in the place of universalism, rights, compassion and talk of rehabilitation has come the vocabulary of the accountant and the prison warder – of 'efficiency', 'markets', discipline and control. There are now no carrots in evidence, only sticks. It is a reversal that not only affects the very poor, but is intended to redraw the lines of advantage and power across the whole class structure of society.

# 2  Impoverishing the poor

The last quarter of the twentieth century in Britain has seen a halting, and then a reversal, of the trends towards greater equality both in income and in wealth, as well as in opportunities for education, health and housing, that had characterised the rest of the century before it. Admittedly these trends to a reduction in inequality had been slow to develop, uneven in pace, and, at the end of the day, very limited in their impact. But they were still taken as evidence of the ability of capitalism to confound its critics – if not of the end of capitalism itself – and in particular of the potential of state intervention to mitigate and perhaps eventually to supersede the inherent inequalities of a market economy.

Since then this trend has been thrown into reverse. In part this is acknowledged to be the result of the economic depression that developed within the global capitalist economy from the 1970s onwards. The impact of this depression and the subsequent restructuring of economies, in terms of mass unemployment and declining relative wages, played a significant part in this reversal. But so too did the activities of the state. It is difficult, probably impossible, to disentangle the two. The adoption by governments, such as in Britain, of tight 'monetarist' policies, even if they did not precipitate at least deepened the impact of economic slump. The pursuit of policies which maintained high levels of unemployment – as, in the words of one British Chancellor of the Exchequer, 'a price well worth paying' for the control of inflation and the confidence of financial institutions – equally prolonged its impact. Both directly, in its role as employer, as provider of benefits and services, and as the body responsible through taxation for deciding who should pay for these, and indirectly, in abolishing restrictions on businesses and capital and removing protection from workers, the state has played a fundamental role in shifting the balance not only of income and wealth, but also of power, back in favour of the rich.

At the same time, private capital has seized the opportunity to restructure its operations: workforces in many companies have been drastically reduced; pay, except for those at the top, has been cut or held back, and work has been subject to intensification through speed-up, longer hours and more managerial control.

It has been and remains a process of enormous significance in which the gains made by working people over the past century whether in civil, social or economic rights have been steadily clawed back on the remarkable premise that they are now a hindrance to progress. It would appear that we are, especially since the collapse of the Soviet empire, now in the midst of a triumphalist capitalism: the leash has been slipped and class barbarism of the most arrogant and brutal forms has once again re-established itself.

The statistics concerning income reveal something of the scale and speed of this shift. In 1979 less than one in ten of the British population had an income below 50 per cent of the average; by 1993 this proportion had risen to one in four (Oppenheim and Harker 1996: 39). While average incomes rose over this period, that of the richest 10 per cent rose the most, by a hefty 65 per cent, while that of the poorest 10 per cent actually fell by 13 per cent (Oppenheim 1997: 23).

The scale – and speed – of this reversal has to be seen in the context of the steady, but slow, reduction in inequality that had characterised the rest of the twentieth century. The Royal Commission on the Distribution of Income and Wealth in its Final Report in 1979 – before it was abolished by the incoming Conservative government – painted a picture 'of substantial inequality in the distribution of income and wealth, but one where those inequalities had been narrowing' (Hills 1996: 1). Between 1979 and 1991, however, this trend was not only thrown into reverse, but rapidly wiped out previous improvements: in the space of a decade the increase in inequality more than doubled the reduction that had taken place since 1949 (Atkinson 1996: 22). As Hills points out:

> What was happening to incomes in the 1980s was very different from what had happened in the previous two decades. In the earlier 18-year period average incomes rose by 35 per cent. For no income group was the increase less than 28 per cent, and for the poorest group incomes rose by over 50 per cent. By contrast, in the 12–13-year period [after 1979] average incomes rose by 36 per cent – as much over this shorter period as over the previous one – but for the bottom seven-tenths of the distribution incomes rose more slowly than the average. Right at the bottom incomes stagnated. Measured

after allowing for housing costs, real incomes at the mid-point of the poorest tenth were 17 per cent lower in 1991/2 than in 1979.

(Hills 1996: 4)

Although many other countries also experienced rises in inequality, nowhere was the increase as great as it was in the UK. In the United States, already one of the most unequal of developed capitalist societies, inequality rose steadily from the mid-1970s, and, measured by the 'gini coefficient', had by 1992 increased by four percentage points; in the shorter period between 1979 and 1991 inequality in the UK rose by almost nine percentage points (Atkinson 1996: 23). Elsewhere, as in Australia or Japan, inequality increased by two to three points, but this trend was by no means universal, and in a number of developed countries inequality remained the same or actually fell over the same period:

> One clear conclusion is that the UK stands out for the sharpness of the rise in recorded income inequality . . . Among the other OECD countries, it is certainly wrong to think in terms of a world-wide trend towards increased income inequality in the 1980s: the upward trend was exhibited to differing degrees in different countries, and was not to be found at all in some countries.
>
> (Atkinson 1996: 23)

Measurements of income inequality are only one aspect of inequality, and are themselves reflections of a number of factors, including not only the operation of capitalism and its labour market (from which most incomes are derived) but also the role of the state in mediating the effects of the market through its systems of taxation and social-security benefits. What is particularly striking about the UK is the shifting significance of these two major factors. Between 1979 and 1985 market incomes polarised rapidly, with the gap growing by five percentage points. This was however offset by the effects of social-security transfers, which reduced the increase in inequality to two points. Over the rest of the decade, however, the activity of the state was to become more important than the market in widening the divide. Between 1985 and 1989, when inequalities of market incomes rose by a further one percentage point, that of gross incomes (i.e. after social-security payments) rose by four points, and disposable income (after taxation) by five points (Atkinson 1996: 43).

This of course in part reflected the Thatcherite celebration of inequality as not only an inevitable but also a necessary condition of a successful capitalist society. The incomes of the rich were to be boosted as an incentive to accumulation and investment. As Brenner noted:

> Capitalists and the wealthy accumulated wealth with such success during the 1980s largely because the state intervened directly to place money in their hands . . . and provided them with an unprecedented array of other politically constituted possibilities to get rich faster through fiscal, monetary and de-regulation policies – all at the expense of the great mass of the people.
>
> (Brenner 1988: 207)

For the poor however the spur of poverty was to be sharpened both by increasing unemployment and changes to the benefit system to increase the incentive to work, to make workers 'less choosy' about what they would and would not do, and to raise productivity. Economic 'success' however (unless defined as the enrichment of a minority) was to prove more elusive.

By the mid-1990s, 20 per cent of working-aged households in Britain had no one in paid work, while of those who were in work over 10 million earned a basic wage less than the Council of Europe decency threshold, and nearly 5 million earned less than half of male median earnings; by 1996 the lowest-paid had fallen further behind the average than at any time since records of wages began in the late nineteenth century (Oppenheim 1997: 23).

These fundamental changes that have reshaped the social and political landscape of British society did not begin just with the election of the Thatcher government in 1979 – although that and successive Conservative governments were to do much to hasten and assist the process of transformation. The symptoms of economic stagnation and crisis were already evident in the mid-1970s: the recession of 1973-5 saw unemployment rise to a post-war record of one million – or nearly 5 per cent of the workforce, compared with an average of less than 2 per cent for the rest of the post-war period – while the cuts in public expenditure introduced by the Labour government between 1975 and 1978 were greater in relative terms than those made by the first Thatcher government that succeeded it (Green 1987). But the roots of crisis lay even further back, in the social and political turmoil of the 1960s, in the historic backwardness of British industrial capitalism during most of the twentieth century, and in particular in the economic, social and political conditions created by the post-war boom itself. For, like all periods of crisis and change, the 1980s were a reaction against what had gone before, as well as laying out the foundations of a changed economic, social and political structure for the future.

In economic terms, the slump of the 1970s, and especially of the first half of the 1980s, international in its scale and devastation, was the inevitable outcome of almost three decades of unprecedented economic growth within the advanced capitalist societies. Inevitable because the logic of capitalist accumulation and development is incapable of maintaining a smooth and uninterrupted trajectory of expansion. This slump followed as inexorably from the boom of the 1950s and 1960s as the slump of the 1920s and 1930s had followed the economic expansion of the first decades of the twentieth century, or as the boom of mid-nineteenth century industrialisation had given way to the first 'great depression' of the 1870s and 1980s. In this context it is not governments which are primarily responsible for economic depression and its consequences, although governments can if they wish do much either to mitigate or to exacerbate the trend. In the final analysis such major economic and social upheavals rest within the dynamics of capitalist production and the social and political conflicts they engender.

It is in such periods that the uncontrolled forces of the market – the anarchy that is capitalist production – are forced to restructure and reorganise themselves. Faced with intense and increasing competition for a collapsing market, employers in the slump of the early 1980s sacked workers and intensified the pressure of work on those who remained. British Steel and British Leyland both cut their workforces by over half; Courtaulds, GKN, Tube Investments, Philips, Dunlop and many other major employers cut theirs by over 40 per cent (*Financial Times* 19 January 1987). Older and less 'efficient' forms of capital were squeezed out, or survive, as many have done in Britain, only by cutting wages and extending the exploitation of their workforces well beyond that of their competitors. With stagnation, surplus capital is released, available through take-overs and mergers to increase and concentrate the power of a small number of giant enterprises and monopolies that will provide the cutting edge and set the standard for the next period of growth. In the intensified competition, new technologies introduce new products and new forms of production, allowing for a more intensive exploitation of labour and advances in productivity and accumulation. The history of capitalism is thus a history of boom and slump, of growth through crisis and destruction. Each major phase in its development has involved a fundamental restructuring: from an agrarian to a manufacturing through various forms of industrial to what many now call a post-industrial society.

The last quarter of the twentieth century has been one such period of major transformation. But it is not only economic forces that have been changed, but also the economic, social and political relationships that go with them. In particular, as in all previous periods of major restructuring, the transformation has had at its heart an assault on the material, social and political gains of labour. The weapon of unemployment was to be one of the major means of carrying this out.

## The unemployment divide

The rapid rise in unemployment in the space of just over two years – from 1.3 million when the Conservative government took office in 1979 to over 3 million by the beginning of 1982, and continuing at post-war record levels ever since – has been one of the most decisive factors in the growing extent and severity of poverty. It has not only affected the incomes and living standards of those unemployed but also, through the intensified competition for jobs and the growing insecurity of many of those who have remained in work, dragged at the wages and living standards of many more. In itself unemployment was to have a major impact on increasing inequality as individuals, families and sometimes whole communities found their major source of income gone. In some cases this was sudden: factory closures announced overnight, and the gates locked the next morning when workers turned up for another day. In others it was a long, slow process of attrition as communities experienced wave upon wave of redundancies.

In the early part of the 1980s at least, the biggest loss was in the older manufacturing and industrial heartlands of the country. The British coal industry, mainly as a consequence of political strategy, as well as revenge, on the part of the Conservative government, was practically destroyed, along with 2 million jobs. In four years, from 1979 to 1983, the number of people employed in manufacturing industry fell by over 1.5 million. Wages in the West Midlands, one of the heartlands of manufacturing, which had stood at 7 per cent above the national average in the 1960s, fell as a consequence to 4 per cent below the average (*Financial Times* 4 April 1984). By 1986 Scotland, Wales, Northern Ireland, the North of England and Yorkshire and Humberside all had one-third fewer workers in manufacturing than they had had in 1979 (*Financial Times* 19 January 1987). The consequences of this devastation on the workers and communities which depended on this employment cannot be over-estimated. In many parts of the country people's sense of identity and security was in part formed by the presence of what were considered to be enduring industries that provided sustenance and security for generations of workers and their families. They were often as much part of the geography as the hills and rivers. Their obliteration in the space of a few years has meant much more than a loss of jobs, as captured in part by this Durham miner describing how life in Easington had changed following the closure of the coal field: 'We are living in a slum clearance area, looking out on boarded up houses. All the kids seem to get for Christmas is a claw hammer and a jemmy. There is no such thing as pride any more' (cited Webster 1998: 3). Those areas bereft of alternative employment were left to wither, lacking any economic foundation and housing only those who could not move. Other changes followed: the jobs that were lost were primarily undertaken by men; those that replaced them, where alternative employment was available, were primarily jobs for women, often at lower rates of pay and in less secure forms of work. According to the director of Bathgate Area Support Enterprise in West Lothian, home to forty new electronics companies that moved in following the collapse of traditional male manufacturing jobs, 'that kind of employment goes to 17-year-old girls or technologists and graduates' (cited *Sunday Times* 27 May 1984). It is the former, however, who are in considerably greater demand, such as at Mitsubishi's video-recorder assembly plant at Livingston, two-thirds of whose workforce is female, with an average age of 18.2 years. There are now 2.3 million fewer men at work, and 1 million more women, than there were twenty years ago (*Independent* 22 November 1993), and the effects both in increasing household poverty and in creating a crisis of male unemployment continue.

With 75 per cent of those unemployed receiving below half of average income (Oppenheim and Harker 1996: 36), unemployment has played a major part in the increase in poverty. But, along with a declining and increasingly restrictive benefit system for the unemployed, it has also meant that the unemployed have come to form a growing proportion not only of the poor in general but of the very poor in particular. In 1979, unemployed people accounted for only one in six of the poorest 10 per cent of the population; by 1992/3 they accounted for one in three (Oppenheim and Harker 1996: 40).

Unemployment is not a static phenomenon but, like the labour market itself, reflects a constant flow of people into and out of work. The headline figures of unemployment thus only reveal a snapshot picture of the numbers unemployed on any one day, while over a longer period considerably more experience its devastating effects. There were in the mid-1990s, on average, about 3.5 million separate new spells of unemployment each year, while over the period 1991–1995 some 10.6 million people experienced unemployment (or, at least, found themselves claiming unemployment benefits, since this is now the official measure of those unemployed): approximately one in three of the labour force (HM Treasury 1997: 5).

The greater the number of people unemployed, the more sluggish is the flow of people back into the labour market, and the more likely people will remain out of work for long periods of time. In 1981 the number of people unemployed for over a year stood at 625,000, or 22 per cent of total unemployment; this figure rose to over 1,238,000, or 43 per cent of the unemployed, by 1987, although it was to fall back again to 25 per cent as overall unemployment fell to the end of the decade, only to rise again to over a million in the recession of the early 1990s (Unemployment Unit 1991 and 1993). For the long-term unemployed, denied the higher rates of benefit available to other long-term claimants of the social-security system, life has been particularly bleak.

Although unemployment rose, and has remained high, at a national level, its effects were concentrated in those parts of the country that were the centres of industrial and manufacturing employment that bore the brunt of the recession of the early 1980s and its shake-out of labour. In 1984 officially recorded unemployment in the Southeast stood at 8.4 per cent, 8.6 per cent in East Anglia and 9.8 per cent in the Southwest of England, while the Northwest recorded levels of 14.7 per cent, the North 16.6 per cent and Northern Ireland 17.7 per cent. In the course of the economic 'boom' of the second half of the 1980s, this structural inequality remained fixed. In April 1988, officially recorded unemployment in both Basingstoke and Crawley (in the Southeast) was less than 3 per cent; in Hartlepool (in the Northeast) and Newquay (in the Southwest) it was over 20 per cent; in parts of Scotland over 25 per cent, while in both Cookstown and Strabane, in Northern Ireland, over 30 per cent of the working population were officially recorded as out of work (Department of Employment 1988).

While such figures confirmed the widely noted divide between the south-eastern parts of England and the rest of the United Kingdom, they also obscure important inequalities within regions, and the persistence of widespread poverty even within areas of apparent affluence. While the Southeast, for example, is by most indicators the most prosperous region in the country, it contains within it – especially in inner London – some of the most severe areas of deprivation. Thus while London's richest 10 per cent of households in 1985 had a gross weekly income of £473, almost £60 a week more than the richest 10 per cent of households in Britain as a whole, the poorest 10 per cent of households in London, with an average income of £47, received £2 each a week less than the average for the poorest 10 per cent for the whole country (Townsend, Corrigan and Kowarzik 1987: 46).

Inequalities of this order – and the poverty associated with them – are not in themselves primarily products of geography. Accidents of geography of course play their part in the siting of coalmines or the existence of facilities for shipbuilding, but the decline, or expansion, of such activities, and the fortunes of the people associated with them, are the products of economic and political forces. In particular they reflect changes in the nature of capitalism, both in the United Kingdom and throughout the world, and the effects of the restructuring of its opera-tions in the face of economic crisis. This much is evident whether we consider the immediate or the long-term history of the United Kingdom. As Doreen Massey has amply demonstrated, 'every major phase in the development of a country's economy has its own geogra-phy' (Massey 1983: 416).

Throughout the post-war boom the structural weakness of those parts of the country based on heavy industry was to continue, the more so as capital employed in the production of ships or steel-making shifted its location to the newly industrialising countries of the world. Yet, for a time, general economic expansion, together with government incentives to new light manufacturing industry to move to the depressed industrial regions, saw some levelling of regional inequalities. Especially during the 1970s, the difference in wage levels between the regions narrowed: from a spread of 20 per cent in 1967, it had shrunk to 9 per cent by 1979 (*Financial Times* 4 April 1984). Already, however, the seeds of a new period of decline, and of new economic and social divisions, had been sown. This time the effects were to be even more dramatic, and, for certain industries such as coal-mining and ship-building, near fatal. A report published in 1995 confirmed the continuation of this trend:

> A broad band of poverty runs from Merseyside into Greater Manchester and parts of South Yorkshire and Tyneside, while a crescent of wealth sweeps up from the south coast and curves around poor areas of inner-city London into East Anglia and the Cotswolds.
>
> (cited *Independent* 1 February 1995)

Thus youth unemployment in Manchester, Liverpool and inner-city London stands at 50 per cent, while in mid-Sussex it is less than 10 per cent. Other reflections of poverty display a similar pattern: a doctor in Richmond, Surrey, has an average of twenty patients with a long-term illness, compared to 600 in Corby or 400 in Easington, while 46 per cent of children in Tower Hamlets in London depend solely on means-tested assistance, compared to 6 per cent in nearby Cambridgeshire. As an article in the *Financial Times* revealed:

Increasingly new and existing companies ... are favouring sites in southern Britain, with a concurrent swing away from urban centres towards rural areas ... The swing towards the rural areas and the south may be taking on an almost unstoppable momentum ... 'The places with economic problems have no chance whatsoever of attracting mobile high technology industry', says Mr Michael Breheny of Reading University. Or, as Peter Ward, Personnel Director of Hewlett Packard (UK) observes, 'It is a case of To Him Who Hath Shall Be Given'.

(*Financial Times* 12 November 1986)

'Places with economic problems' – for which we can read most of the major conurbations – found themselves in the reverse of this trap. As the *Observer* reported:

The odds are overwhelmingly stacked against a northern working man [sic] moving south, however skilled and however strong his motivation. If he has a council house, with whom does he exchange it? If he owns a house, how can he sell it for anything like the value of a home in the south? Company after company told of the abortive recruiting drives in the north. They could find the men they wanted, but, often after a few miserable months in a bedsit searching every night for a family home that could be afforded on a working wage however lavish or slavish the overtime – the workers would trail home defeated for an indefinite future on the dole.

(*Observer* 11 January 1987)

## The earnings divide

In 1943 the *Times* warned of the dangers of the growing movement in support of a government-maintained policy of 'full employment':

Unemployment is not a mere accidental blemish in a private enterprise economy. On the contrary, it is part of the essential mechanism of the system, and has a definite function to fill. The first function of unemployment (which has always existed in open or disguised forms) is that it maintains the authority of master over man. The master has normally been in the position to say 'If you don't want the job, there are plenty of others who do.' When the man can say: 'If you don't want to employ me, there are plenty of others who will', the situation is radically altered.

(cited Beveridge 1945: 195)

The alteration of this relationship during the immediate post-war years of relatively full employment provided the basis for an increase in wages and standards of living, as well as for a narrowing of inequalities between the highest- and the lowest-paid. From the 1960s until the early 1970s real wages rose uniformly across the whole working population, while the wages of the lowest-paid actually increased relative to others during the period of the Labour government's Social Contract. From the late 1970s, however, as unemployment began to rise, so too did inequalities in earnings, and during the 1980s the differential sharpened considerably. According to an Incomes Data Services report, the net pay of company chief executives increased by 645 per cent between 1979 and 1994, that of senior directors by 579 per cent (*Independent* 4 March 1994). By 1992 median wages had increased by 35 per cent over their 1979 levels, those of the richest tenth by over 50 per cent, but those of the lowest-paid stagnated, never to recover their position of the mid-1970s.

Government policy was to play a significant part in this polarisation. In contrast to the general encouragement of 'initiative' and 'enterprise', swingeing tax cuts and grotesque salary increases to the already highly paid as an 'incentive' to business, specific steps were taken to remove protection against wage cuts from the lowest-paid. The Fair Wages Resolution, established in 1891 to require private firms working on government contracts to provide levels of pay and conditions similar to those in other comparable firms, was abolished in 1983, paving the way for pay reductions for low-paid workers especially in the public sector, as hospitals and local authorities were forced by legislation to put an increasing amount of the work undertaken in areas such as cleaning, catering and security out to competitive tender. The lowest-paid were again targeted for action when the protection of the minimum wage levels set by national Wages Councils was removed first from half a million young workers under the age of 21, and then from all low-paid workers when the Wages Councils were abolished.

Before their abolition the Wages Councils set minimum rates in only a limited and specified number of particularly low-paid occupations, and the actions of the dwindling number of Wage Inspectors were scarcely draconian: in 1985 35 per cent of employers visited were found to be illegally underpaying their workers, yet only two were prosecuted (*Financial Times* 29 September 1986). Although big business in particular remained ambivalent about the state regulation of the wages that the Wages Councils represented – some fearing a return to the cutthroat competition that had sparked their introduction 100 years earlier – support for their abolition was nevertheless forthcoming. As for the effects on the already low-paid, Sir Terence Beckett, Director General of the employers' organisation the CBI, thought 'such concerns, where legitimate, should be met through the social security system, and not through pay. An employer can only pay the rate for the job' (*Financial Times* 23 May 1983).

Assisted by such governmental actions, the 'rate for the job' declined. By 1995, half of all jobs previously covered by Wage Council protection were paying less than the minimum wage would otherwise have been, while over 75 per cent of workers in hairdressing, hotels and catering, shops and the garment trade earned less than the level of means-tested assistance for a family with two children (*Guardian* 30 August 1995). According to the Low Pay Unit, four out of ten full-time workers and three-quarters of part-time workers now earn less than the Council of Europe 'decency threshold' (set at two-thirds of average earnings). Although women make up the majority of part-time low-paid workers (4.5 million, compared to 800,000 men), the most dramatic increase since 1979 has been in the proportion of full-time men in low-paid work, which increased from 15 to 30 per cent. What this has produced has been a growing polarisation in wage levels. Average pay rises from 1980 to 1993 were £94,000 for the top 1 per cent of taxpayers, and just over £4,000 for the bottom half of the population. Compared with higher-paid workers, the lower-paid have seen their earnings fall: for both male and female full-time workers the ratio fell from over 40 per cent in 1979 to just over 30 per cent by 1994 (Low Pay Unit 1994).

One consequence of the lowering of wage levels has been a rise in the number of people with more than one job: the number with second jobs, for example, doubling since 1983 to 1.3 million (Office for National Statistics 1997). It has also put increasing pressure on families for both partners in a couple to go out to work. The number of dual-income households has increased significantly, giving rise to increased attention to and concern over the division between what has been caricatured as 'work-rich' and workless households. Certainly, the number of households without anyone in paid employment has risen, reaching one in five by the early 1990s, many caught in the trap by which means-tested benefits penalise the poor. But to characterise the remainder as 'work-rich' obscures the fact that large numbers are quite literally overworked, while the financial returns of this development are deeply unequal. Hewlett notes that in the USA, 'the average worker is now at work 163 hours a year more than in 1967, which adds up to an extra month of work annually. In a similar vein, time spent on the job in the UK increased by two hours a week during the 1980s' (Hewlett 1993: 2). We now live in a society where for many the fear of losing employment means that there has been a massive increase in exploitation, as if hours spent on the job were some indication of one's commitment and indispensability.

While some families need two, three or even more jobs simply to survive, often at great expense to health and family life, others reap the benefits of dual incomes in greatly increased consumption. The division of dual-income households according to social class is a crucial dimension of this phenomenon. The rise in the number of women working, from one-quarter of the workforce in 1966 to one-half, has had a marked impact on inequalities between working households: 65 per cent of professional and managerial women work full-time, and only 17 per cent part-time, while amongst unskilled manual women only 8 per cent work full-time, while 55 per cent work part-time. In 1994 the average earnings of full-time professional women were £400 per week, those of part-time manual women less than £70 (*Guardian* 27 September 1995). Higher incomes for some has meant an increased demand for services; with this has gone a rapid growth in the number of low-paid jobs to service the whims and needs of those with the money to spend.

Britain has emerged from the 1980s, by European and even by global comparison, as a relatively low-paid economy. This, together with the reduced rights and protection afforded to British workers, has made it an attractive, if often temporary, place for investment by transnational corporations producing goods for the European market. The traffic, however, has not only been one way. As Paul Webster reported:

> French police are investigating a cross-Channel traffic in cheap labour. Police said that at least 14 cases of exploited British work gangs were under investigation in the Pas de Calais, the Lille area and Normandy. Most were similar to a case at Argentan, Normandy, where a British subcontractor, Robert Butcher, was fined more than £20,000 and given a year's suspended jail sentence for flouting French and European labour laws. Mr. Butcher was accused of failing to provide social security and pay slips, and failing to pay taxes. He told the magistrate that it was easy to find jobless men ready to work for 300 francs a day (£33) because of the 'British social climate'. He recruited in pubs, and toured sites in France offering workers for hire. His methods were 'common practice' in Britain. The prosecution claims that the use of British workers undercut the price of subcontracted work by 60 per cent.
>
> (*Guardian* 3 December 1996)

During the Thatcher era the unemployed were told to 'get on their bikes' and to 'price themselves back into work'. The consequence was declining wages for those at the lower end of the labour market. It is a policy that has continued in the 1990s, with Britain's international competitiveness sought on the basis of the cheapness of its labour. According to the New Labour government, 'lack of flexibility in real wages has been a long-standing problem of the British economy' (HM Treasury 1997: 17). Although inequalities in pay now exceed the level of 100 years ago, and although 45 per cent of new entrants to the labour market can expect to earn less than one-quarter of median earnings (Gregg and Wadsworth 1995), this is apparently not enough. Further 'flexibility' is also needed 'in relative wages . . . to exploit the new opportunities available' (ibid.): hence the prospect of an even wider gap between top and bottom. But the government also argues that the economy 'also needs real wage flexibility' – with the result that all wages can fall – 'so that wage setting processes are responsive to the level of unemployment' (ibid.).

Unemployment is now set to be maintained at levels that continue to exert a downward pressure on wages. Government and other economists, who have for years invented 'explanations' for unemployment, few of which have ever got near the truth, have now adopted the Non-Accelerating Inflation Rate of Unemployment (NAIRU) as a guiding principle of economic policy. This predicts a minimum and necessary number of unemployed as a target for government policy to maintain economic equilibrium. Curiously, 'the NAIRU cannot be observed and is very difficult to measure . . . It must therefore be inferred from observed inflation and unemployment data, and other labour market indicators' (HM Treasury 1997: 4). Yet, despite the difficulty of establishing its existence, this standard forms a fundamental principle of government policy, signifying its intention to use unemployment and the unemployed as a means of regulating wages.

Despite its consequences, the low-pay strategy adopted by the Thatcher government and continued by its successors is itself by no means assured of success. Still less is there evidence that 'getting people into work' – however minimal the return – is a stepping-stone to a career out of poverty. As the Treasury's own report states:

> People on low wages have tended to stay on low wages: 48 per cent of men in the bottom tenth remained there one year later, and of the remainder only 20 per cent moved up the distribution. (The rest have dropped out of the earnings distribution altogether.) Even after three years, 26 per cent remain in the bottom tenth . . . Of the men who were in the bottom quarter of the earnings distribution in

1991, half were still there in 1994, 13 per cent were out of work altogether, while only 6 per cent had ascended to the top half.

(HM Treasury 1997: 9)

When the head of the world's largest cleaning company, ISS, after losing a £2.5 million contract at Heathrow Airport to a lower bidder, criticised low pay levels in Britain as 'uneconomic and socially divisive' (cited *Guardian* 23 September 1994), he expressed a long-standing concern of a section of British capital, in particular of big business, about the effects of a 'competitive' economy whose competition is based solely on the cheapest possible production. In the short term low wages may offer a competitive benefit, if not to those who earn them, then at least to those who pay them, although such a strategy is at the cost of mounting individual and social distress. In the longer term it offers no possibility of economic growth, other than through a continuation of the same downward spiral.

> Industries which come to rely upon cheap labour provide a way in which inefficient producers and obsolete technologies can survive and compete. Firms become caught in low productivity traps from which they have little incentive to escape. When these firms are subjected to competition from more efficient firms, with improved technology and products, their only hope of survival is to reduce wages further. In periods of full employment this is only possible to a limited extent because [of] the existence of alternative job opportunities for their workers . . . In periods of high unemployment, however, this discipline is lifted. The most vulnerable in the labour market become increasingly vulnerable and the ease by which their wages and conditions of work can be further depressed provides the basis for the competitive survival of inefficient producers . . . [This] further reduces the incentive to invest and innovate and builds up reliance on low pay and casualised employment as the only means of survival.
>
> (Brosnan and Wilkinson 1987: 19–20)

## The employment divide

During the 1980s and into the 1990s the conditions of the labour market changed dramatically in Britain, leading to a growing polarisation not only between those in work and those out of work but also amongst those who remained in employment. The impact of sustained high levels of unemployment was felt not only by those dismissed or denied the opportunity of a job. As Ron Todd, then senior negotiator for the Transport and General Workers' Union, saw it a year after the Tories' first election victory, 'we have three million on the dole and another twenty five million scared to death' (cited Beynon 1983: 4). The fear – and the threat – of unemployment became a weapon in the hands of employers keen to reduce wages and working conditions, to discipline their workforces, and to reverse what they saw as the unjustified advances that working people had made in the post-war decades of full employment and trade-union strength. As one management consultant advised:

> We have an opportunity that will last for two or three years, then the unions will get themselves together again and the government, like all governments, will run out of steam. So grab it now . . . We have had a pounding, and we are all fed up with it. I think it would be fair to say it is almost vengeance.
>
> (cited Beynon 1983: 15)

This 'window of opportunity' was, however, to last much longer than he had anticipated. Through the rest of the decade, and into the 1990s, British capitalism was dramatically to redefine its relationship with its employees, not only to demand, and often achieve, a lowering of wages, but also to bring about significant changes in the structure and processes of work and in the imposition of new and more arbitrary forms of discipline.

Part of this transformation, with consequences for the poverty and increased insecurity of millions, has been changes in the organisation of work. According to Charles Leadbetter:

> A transformation is taking place in the shape of the UK workforce. The predominance of secure full-time jobs is giving way under pressure of high unemployment, weakened trade unions, rising female unemployment and removal of labour market restrictions, yielding a fluid mixture, which includes temporary workers and whose who work part-time, at home or for themselves.
>
> (*Financial Times* 27 February 1987)

Writing as economics editor of the *Financial Times*, John Lloyd noted in the mid-1980s how:

> The change that has had the most effect on Britain over the past

decade – the rapid rise in unemployment – is now less important as a continuing process than the shifts within the employed workforce . . . The composition, skills level, mobility and hours worked by those who have jobs are being forced into new moulds.

(*Financial Times* 13 June 1986)

These new moulds have come to shape a labour market that is itself increasingly polarised. According to one report, 'companies are restructuring their work forces into an inner core of workers with relatively secure employment who are essential to operations, and an outer periphery of staff such as temporary workers, whose employment can be ended easily' (*Financial Times* 24 September 1985). Employers have sought to reduce the size of their permanent workers to those who are essential, whose skills are in high demand, or in whom substantial investment in the form of training has been made. For such workers – primarily white-collar staff, but also a number of skilled manual workers – firms often operate their own internal recruitment and promotion systems, offering a range of fringe benefits from cars to private health insurance and much higher degrees of job security.

The peripheral workforce, on the other hand, encompasses a wide range of employment conditions, including part-time, temporary, casual and self-employment. Its growth, with two-thirds of all new jobs created in the 1990s being temporary or part-time, reflects a desire on the part of employers to reduce reliance on full-time permanent, and often unionised, workers, and instead to employ workers – where possible – according to weekly, daily and even hourly needs. The preference of employers to take on young or married women, often new to the world of paid employment, has also contributed to the gendering of this peripheral workforce. In 1987 the Department of Employment produced the first official national estimate of the size of this core and peripheral workforce, showing that while the permanent workforce had fallen by 1.02 million, or 6 per cent, between 1981 and 1985, the peripheral workforce had grown by 1.15 million, or 16 per cent (*Financial Times* 5 February 1987), to make up one-third of those in employment. The fact that the majority of job losses occurred in the early part of this period, at a time of recession, while the 'new' jobs increased as the economy began to recover, indicated a trend amongst employers to seek economic expansion primarily by taking on part-time or temporary workers rather than full-time and permanent ones.

In conditions of large-scale unemployment, employers often had a free hand to change work contracts and conditions, with little prospect of effective opposition. As the divisional organiser for the engineering union in the Northwest of England noted, 'We've been taken to the cleaners by companies who are trying to casualise their workforce' (cited *Financial Times* 13 January 1983). Some employers did this directly, sacking permanent full-time staff only to offer them re-employment on a part-time or casual basis. Thus early in 1983 the British Steel Corporation sacked 630 workers in Teesside, offering to take them back on short-term contracts as and when work was available. As a *Sunday Times* report noted, 'northern employers with their backs to the wall are now well aware that there is a vast pool of unemployed labour available at the drop of a hat for a week or two's work' (*Sunday Times* 30 January 1983). Other employers have put their workers onto short-term or casual contracts simply to avoid the legal obligations that follow from full-time employment, even though in many cases these 'temporary' contracts are annually renewed, or 'casual' workers find themselves working longer hours than permanent ones. More generally, firms have sought to slim down their own operations, using subcontractors and employment agencies to supply much of the labour needed, for example, in cleaning, catering or secretarial services previously employed within the firm itself. This secondary or peripheral workforce acts as a buffer against market fluctuations, allowing employers to increase or decrease output without having to bear the costs of redundancy payments or carry large fixed overheads. The managing director of one large manufacturing company expressed a common reluctance to take on permanent workers like this: 'I'll go on overtime first, and then on extended deliveries rather than get caught again' (cited *Financial Times* 4 April 1984). It has also been for many a way of avoiding the build-up of industrial-relations disputes that had been a consequence of expanding their workforces during the post-war boom. According to the commercial director of Livingston Development Corporation, the attraction of such workers, especially those entering paid employment for the first time, is that they are 'uncontaminated', a point spelled out by a director of the computer software company Ferranti Infographics: 'This area has been notoriously highly unionised over the years and employers tend to think that if you have been in a union environment, it will have worked its way into you' (cited *Financial Times* 18 January 1988).

The casualisation of the labour market, with its increased insecurity, is a trend that has continued to grow. In 1961 only 4 per cent of workers were employed on a part-time basis; by the mid-1980s this had risen to 22 per cent of all workers, and 30 per cent of workers in the service industries (*Financial Times* 3 September 1987). Today, 44 per cent of all workers are in either part-time, temporary or self-employment (HM

Treasury 1997). As one employer remarked, 'we are creating a two-class structure, with one of the classes being like guest workers' (cited *Financial Times* 4 April 1984).

The increased casualisation of the labour market and the growing insecurity facing many of those in work has compounded the material impact of poverty. According to one report, 'people in insecure jobs are experiencing levels of psychological distress close to those of the unemployed' (*Financial Times* 10 July 1994), with consequent effects on the break-up of marriages and relationships. But stress, like the poverty with which it is most closely associated, is also a killer. According to Ian Banks of the British Medical Association, suicide is 'the big new killer of men and is shockingly popular – it has doubled in the last ten years. The one clear cause is uncertainty at work' (cited Pilger 1998: 80). In similar vein, the *Times* (22 February 1995) reported that up to 1.7 million working days are lost to work-related stress each year, amounting to an estimated 40 per cent of the £25 billion lost annually due to absence through ill-health. It is salutary to note that despite these facts being 'known', so little action is taken to counteract these trends.

## A servile workforce

'We've got to somehow get it into people's minds', argued Lord Young, the minister charged by Margaret Thatcher with overseeing the removal of employment protection and, with that, the hope of creating new jobs, 'that you don't equate service with being servile.' The proportion of workers employed in service industries has grown steadily, from less than half in 1964, to 58 per cent in 1978 and 63 per cent by 1983. As a long-term trend this is common to all advanced capitalist societies; in the short term, the collapse of manufacturing in the early 1980s saw a loss both of jobs and of output, and although output was eventually to recover its previous levels, the number of jobs in manufacturing never did. Although service-sector employment also fell slightly during the first recession of the 1980s, the fall was nowhere near as great, and since then its expansion has continued as an enduring feature of the economy.

As a category of employment, the service sector is a huge generalisation, encompassing those who work as cleaners or shop assistants as well as those who work as financiers or commodity brokers. While some celebrate the growth of service-sector employment as signalling an end to dangerous or dirty jobs, the reality is very different. For many, and certainly for the fastest-growing sectors of employment, service-sector jobs are more often low-paid, boring and mundane. According to one account:

Dean Smith, 31, earns £3.20 an hour. This is 20p more than when he started at his company nearly three years ago – and 70p an hour more than many of the jobs advertised where he lives. Mr Smith is a security guard at a leisure complex outside Manchester. He gets no overtime and works up to 60 hours a week, mostly evenings . . . Although Mr Smith lives in Manchester, he is often sent to other complexes in Preston or Chester. He is given an extra hour's pay, but not travelling expenses. In his last pay cheque, he took home £93 after tax for 34.75 hours. Money is deducted for his 15 minute tea break. 'The worst thing about the job is the unsocial hours. I have to work every weekend. The other day they made me come all the way in to show this lad around on my night off – they paid me for one hour at £3.20, but if I say anything they'll just cut my hours down', he said. 'You do get holiday pay, but they calculate it depending on how many hours you've worked in the previous 12 weeks, so they cut your hours down deliberately'. For last year's ten day holiday he was paid for 19 hours. 'People don't realise what sort of life we have to lead. In my area you see jobs advertised for £2.50 an hour. The employers know you can claim family credit and they will just cut your wages', he said. 'I would feel differently about my employers if I got paid more – as it is they make you feel like you're not worth anything, that you're just a commodity'.

(*Independent* 9 September 1996)

In important ways the growth in service-sector employment is not simply the consequence of a maturing industrial economy, but also reflects an increasingly polarised society. The market research firm Mintel's British Lifestyle Report for 1994 forecasts growing income inequality until at least the end of the century; as a consequence, 'on the one hand there is an increasing demand for luxury goods and services, while on the other a growing proportion of households only have sufficient income for staple products and necessities' (cited *Independent* 1 February 1994). The polarisation of income and jobs has meant that those with money to spend increasingly employ nannies, cooks, cleaners and other household assistance in order to enable themselves to go out to work, while equally depending upon low-paid service workers to satisfy their demands for leisure. The Director of the US Bureau of Labor Statistics summed this up when he noted:

Much of the demand for services has to do with the nature of our culture and the changes we are going through. The large number of two-income families has increased wealth and demand for services like fast food, entertainment and vacations.

(*Businessweek* July 1984)

The growth of the fast-food industry is a prime example of this trend. During the 1970s it was one of the fastest-growing areas of employment in the United States economy: the increase alone in the number of new workers employed in that decade exceeding the total employment in basic steel-making. Like many other developments in leisure and entertainment – of which eating, like shopping, has increasingly been made a part – its growth reflects not only increasing disposable income for some, but also changing household composition and cultural patterns. As more people live alone (24 per cent of households in 1983 compared with 11 per cent in 1961), and as more married women have left the sole occupation of housewife to become wage-earners as well (an increase from 26 per cent to 57 per cent between 1951 and 1981), so the demand for 'fast food' in a fast-paced economy has grown. The trend is also one which embodies the polarisation between those who consume and those who produce such services. In a radio interview in 1985, Martin Price, the manager of a dynamic high-tech advanced telecommunications company in Stevenage, put it like this:

Only by the success of companies like ours will the economy set itself for the others to follow. And it's in these other sectors that there will be more opportunities for the lower skilled people. We're talking straightforward economics here. IDEC, like other companies in Stevenage, is generating wealth. That wealth goes into Stevenage and people have it to spend. I bet you we sell more Wimpeys in Stevenage than McDonalds sell their hamburgers in Worksop. And, of course, to sell more hamburgers, more people will need to be employed to prepare them and sell them. That makes more jobs of that kind.

(BBC Radio 4 Analysis, 4 November 1985)

'More jobs of that kind' – with fast-food outlets in Britain growing by the mid-1980s at 15 per cent a year (*Financial Times* 9 August 1986) – means more low-paid, insecure, casual and part-time work. The big multiple fast-food chains that have proliferated in Britain since the 1970s encapsulate important trends in the growth of such services. Overwhelmingly non-union (if not explicitly anti-union) they depend upon a workforce that is predominantly young and low-paid. McDonalds, for example, in 1985 employed 12,000 people in Britain, 85 per cent of them on a part-time basis, 75 per cent under the age of 21, at minimum wages of £1.60 an hour (*Financial Times* 28 June 1985). That they were able to do so was a reflection of high levels of youth unemployment, but also of the drive in the leading sectors of the service economy towards high levels of capital investment and automation (the average Wimpy restaurant in Britain, for example, requiring an investment of £450,000) that reduces workers' tasks to a series of routine and repetitive motions for which little training or skill is required, and which makes such workers easily, and frequently, replaceable. 'It was horrible', recalls one 19-year-old, 'slave labour. They used to pay you a pittance for all that work. You were like a robot, a link in a chain. It was like . . . it was like a communist regime' (*Observer* 23 November 1986).

Leisure services and tourism, along with the financial-services sector, have since the 1980s been the fastest-growing sectors of the British economy. Their expansion reflects and compounds the growing economic and social divide. On the one hand they provide a supply of insecure and low-paid casual work as waiters, hotel chambermaids or the countless other service jobs that are available to the poor; on the other they have produced the phenomenon of highly-paid brokers and financial speculators with money to spend on services that the poor are employed to provide.

The last two and a half decades have seen new cleavages emerge within cities and urban conurbations as jobs in the manufacturing sector have haemorrhaged and new employment (where it has been created at all) has not gone to those who have been made jobless. In the sixteen big cities outside of London, for example, there has been up to a one-third increase in higher-level white-collar jobs (Webster 1998), with a resulting gentrification of many inner-city areas. New, and expensive, developments of luxury flats and apartments, entertainment and shopping complexes, such as those constructed in the former dockland areas of London or Liverpool, symbolise this contrast. Sited on areas of previous working-class employment – now gone for ever – they flaunt their opulence often no more than a stone's throw away from areas of extreme poverty and neglect. The long-established North–South divide has thus been compounded by what the Henley Centre for Forecasting describes as 'massive differences in economic vitality between localities right across the country' in which 'winners and losers live side by side'. Within the cities it sees a 'growing band of people who gain no benefit from the regeneration of city centres and whose fortunes are generally declining. The co-existence of increasing prosperity and expanding poverty clearly raises important questions about social cohesion. This polarisation . . . creates the potential for the spread of no-go areas' (*Independent* 17 June 1994). As Campbell (1993) noted in her study of the riots that rocked some of these areas in the early 1990s, what were once homes to thousands of employed manual workers have been transformed into abandoned places with no or little prospect of secure employment. Many, such as the Aylesbury estate in London (where Tony Blair made a symbolic visit shortly after his election as Prime Minister in 1997) are left as little more than open prisons (Pilger 1998: 79).

For some of the dispossessed who look on at these new developments there is sometimes employment to be found. But it is employment of a different sort from that which has been lost: more often for women than for men, more often part-time than full-time, it is predominantly low-paid servicing work meeting the needs of a middle class that is either new to the area or that lives outside the city and drives in on fast new road systems – bypassing the eyesores of inner-city dereliction – to spend an evening's leisure before speeding out again to the suburbs. For others who stand and look, these new developments – like the mushrooming shopping centres and malls, the wine bars and private gyms – represent a spectacle of consumption usually beyond reach. Few can afford to buy the designer goods and luxuries on display, and drift through looking in windows at goods they can never afford. As Victor Keegan observed, 'never in the history of the world have they [the rich] been present in such quantities and in such flamboyant contrast with the poor as now' (*Guardian* 22 July 1996).

## Changing social security

As if increased job insecurity, stagnant or falling wages and the misery of unemployment were not enough, the immiseration created by the labour market has been added to by the creation of a meaner, more controlled and more punitive state benefit system.

That the social-security system has been made meaner just as the conditions of the labour market have worsened is of course no accident. Social security has never been just a system for maintaining those without sufficient income; throughout its history this aim has been over-ridden by the perceived need to fashion benefits according to the requirements of the labour market. So it is that, except for those with children, for whom a low-wage subsidy was introduced in the 1970s, people in work are not entitled to claim benefit, no matter how great their need. The principle of less eligibility entombed in the 1834 Poor Law Amendment Act – that the relief of poverty should always be made less attractive than the condition of the low-paid – lives on, driven relentlessly downwards by the deteriorating conditions of the labour market itself.

During the 1980s the social-security system was to be used to buttress the offensive against employment and job security. As firms shed labour and sought to change working practices for those who remained, the effectiveness of the weapon, and the threat, of unemployment was determined in part by the fate of the unemployed. This put them at the forefront of government policy, to be joined in the 1990s by the spectre of single mothers on benefit and other groups of the 'undeserving' poor as state benefits came to be used to buttress not only a failing labour market but also the perceived decline of the family and moral order.

At something under 15 per cent of all social-security expenditure, unemployment-related benefits are, in financial terms, a relatively small target. The much bigger issue of pensions, consuming by far the largest part of social-security spending, was and has remained politically a much more difficult target to attack. Although legislation introduced in 1980 broke the link between pensions (and other benefits) and earnings, so that state pensions have ever since continually failed to keep pace with the general rise in the standard of living, proposals to privatise at least part of the state pensions scheme, or to take more radical action to prune the largest part of the social-security budget, came to naught. State pensions, although falling yearly in relative value, nevertheless constitute a bedrock of financial provision for all retired people, on which middle- and some working-class people have built additional private or occupational provision.

Those retired without additional private pensions or savings have found themselves left only able to claim means-tested assistance. Like other claimants of means-tested benefits, including the vast majority of the unemployed and of single parents, and anyone not in work whose income falls below the minimal level provided, they have experienced a system which has become increasingly constrained, less responsive to individual need and more punitive in its actions. Although successive governments have made much of the need to restrain the growth of the social-security budget, the effects have not been felt equally by all claimants. As the composition of the poorest has changed – partly as a result of state policy itself – and as the numbers of the poor have increased, so those left dependent on the state's minimum means-tested benefits have borne the brunt of 'reform'.

Although both the proportion of national income redistributed through the social-security system and the level of benefit paid to individual claimants in Britain lags far behind that of other comparable countries, successive governments have argued that the growing cost of social-security provision in Britain has become unsustainable. The assault on the state benefit system that has characterised government policy since the beginning of the 1980s has, however, to be seen as more than simply a response to the rising cost of social security and an attempt to reduce or restrain public expenditure. Indeed, measured by those objectives, such a policy has been spectacularly unsuccessful. Despite a succession of cuts in the level of most benefits, and despite the imposition of stricter conditions for the receipt of many of them, the social-security budget has continued to rise. Given the sustained high levels of unemployment, and the massive growth of poverty and inequality, this is hardly surprising. But what the rhetoric of public expenditure constraints conceals is that the costs of cuts and changes in the social-security system have fallen disproportionately on the poorest. This is despite official insistence that the reform of social security is intended to concentrate help on those who need it most. The 1992 Conservative Party election manifesto, for example, after noting a 40 per cent increase in real expenditure on social security, went on: 'This extra help is more clearly focused on those groups with the greatest needs' (cited Piachaud 1997: 76). As Piachaud demonstrates, however, although expenditure on benefits increased significantly during the 1980s, the proportion going to the poorest 20 per cent actually fell between 1979 and 1995 by nearly 15 per cent. The extra spending on social security that took place went to other groups (except the richest), most notably to boost the falling incomes of the next poorest 20 per cent (half of whose income by 1995 came from benefits) and the middle 20 per cent (one-quarter of whose income was made up of state benefits). In all cases, however, this increased expenditure failed to prevent the total income of these groups declining as a proportion of average income. In part, of course, what this reveals is that 'need' in the context of social security is a matter of political definition. It is not, nor ever has been, based simply on the objective situation of particular individuals or groups of the poor. Whether people are seen as in 'need' of help has also been a judgement about whether they deserve help, and this has been a matter both of political expediency and moral judgement.

The 1986 Social Security Act, although announced by the Secretary of State as forming the most fundamental review of social security since Beveridge, was in effect to concentrate its attention on means-tested benefits. The new system of Income Support which it introduced to replace the old system of Supplementary Benefit was to confirm the 'mass role' of means-testing in the social-security system. Means-tested assistance was no longer to be, as the post-war reconstruction of social security had intended, an exceptional provision tailored to the needs of those who fell through the system of universal insurance benefits provided as a right regardless of means. It was now to be refashioned as the major source of benefit for a large part of the population.

Central to this was the question of the extent to which such a system could, or should, tailor assistance to the circumstances of individual claimants. Such an aim had, at least in theory, been a central rationale of the Supplementary Benefit system and its predecessors. Where Beveridge had envisaged a social-security system in which the vast majority of claimants would receive a standard rate of insurance benefit as of right, means-tested assistance would allow a fine tuning of help both for those who failed to qualify for insurance-based benefit and for those whose needs were 'exceptional'. In practice, however, means-tested assistance functioned to allow the basic rates of benefit (both its own and those of the main insurance-based scheme) to be kept extremely low; those without other means would qualify for extra assistance, while the exceptional needs of individual claimants such as the disabled or the chronic sick could be met through additional payments administered through a complex process of investigation at the discretion of officials.

These additional payments thus formed the 'safety-valve' of the whole social-security system. In 1978 the Labour government, amidst official concern about the growing number of additional payments that were being made (itself a reflection of the low basic rate of benefit), announced a review of their operation. The results of this were to be taken up by the Conservative government that replaced it, and in 1980 the Thatcher government's first Social Security Act worked decisively in the attempt to halt their growth. The discretionary powers that had previously been allowed to Supplementary Benefit officials to vary the weekly rate of benefit (a power that had also been used in certain cases to reduce benefit) or to make exceptional one-off payments were now to be ended and replaced by detailed regulations which circumscribed the specific conditions under which particular claimants could be allowed, for example, the cost of a second-hand cooker or furniture. Even then these more restricted additions were payable only, according to the regulations, 'if, in the opinion of the benefit officer, such a payment is the only means by which serious damage or serious risk to the health or safety of any member of the assessment unit may be prevented'.

The role of individual and local discretion, as opposed to centralised rules and regulations, has been a constant quandary in the history of the social-security system. On the one hand the state has sought to impose central control, while on the other it has feared, in the words of the 1834 Poor Law Report, that without a local administration the remoteness of decision-making in Whitehall would mean that 'vigilance and economy would be relaxed; that the workhouses would be allowed to breed an hereditary population and would cease to be objects of terror'. In the early nineteenth century the solution was to be a locally administered system, under elected Boards of Guardians, guided by a central inspectorate. By 1934, with the extension of the franchise beyond the property-owning classes, the refusal of a number of local Boards of Guardians to follow central government regulations (for example, in the imposition of the means test or the payment of benefit to strikers) led to the centralisation of administration in the Unemployment Assistance Board that was in 1948 to become the National Assistance Board. But officials still retained the power to vary levels of benefit or to make exceptional payments. In 1968 these powers passed to the newly formed Supplementary Benefits Commission, where they were to become a focal point for claimants' organisations, mobilised to increase the level of benefit payments. It was in this context that the Thatcher government's first Social Security Act was passed; one Conservative MP summed up the context succinctly: 'There is far too much talk about rights,' argued Peggy Fenner during the House of Commons debate, 'whether they be welfare rights or the right to withdraw one's labour.'

The impact of the new regulations was to produce an immediate drop in the number of single payments made, from 1.2 million in 1978 to 800,000 by 1981. Yet the regulations, stringent though they were, were also to make public, and official rather than discretionary, the conditions under which such payments could be made. In a situation of increasing poverty they were once again to become the focus of claims. By 1984 the number of successful claims for additional payments had increased to 3 million; compared to less than one-quarter in 1981, now over half of all claimants (and over three-quarters of non-pensioner claimants) received an 'exceptional' single payment. Requiring the work of 2,500 officials, and constituting 21 per cent of all social-security appeals, single payments had become 'a considerable cause of friction between claimants and staff'. Accordingly the 1986 White Paper announced, 'The Government considers that routine provision of one-off payments in principle open to all claimants, is no longer appropriate' (Department of Health and Social Security 1986: 23).

The rationale for the reform of the Supplementary Benefit system, and its replacement by Income Support, was that 'the present scheme offers a false prospectus in attempting to deal with extremely large numbers of claimants as if each individual's precise circumstances can be examined in detail' (Department of Health and Social Security 1986: 19). With over 4 million people now dependent on it, and with no intention of reversing the drift of social-security provision away from insurance towards a mass role for means-tested benefits, the system would now be 'simplified': 'the aim will be to give claimants a reasonable level of help rather than to provide in detail for every variation in individual circumstances' (Department of Health and Social Security 1986: 23).

This 'reasonable level of help', however, was not to be dictated by what people needed, nor by what the country could afford. Indeed, 'it is doubtful whether an attempt to establish an objective standard of adequacy would be useful' (Department of Health and Social Security 1986: 20), and although the White Paper stated that 'the level of help for those on Supplementary Benefit cannot be isolated from consideration of both the returns and rewards that are available to people in society in general', it is clear that it did not have in mind the rapidly growing wealth and income of the minority who were benefiting from the government's cuts in taxation or the changing conditions of the labour market. The comparison, on the contrary, was to be made with the working poor:

> The rapid growth in payments in the last few years has raised considerable questions of fairness with those not on benefit. The availability of payments for those on benefit stands in sharp contrast to the position faced by many others, on what may not be very different levels of disposable income, who have to budget for such items.
>
> (Department of Health and Social Security 1986: 22)

Proposing a system of 'rough justice' in which there would be both 'winners and losers' (although the latter were significantly to outnumber the former), the weekly additions to benefit achieved by some claimants were to be replaced, at no additional cost, by a standard premium paid to the disabled, pensioners and those with children. The unemployed, in their own right, were to be excluded. In terms of single one-off payments, the White Paper proposed 'a more effective and responsive system' (Department of Health and Social Security 1986: 32) that would be known as the Social Fund. In the place of detailed regulations would be a system 'administered by DHSS local offices on a discretionary basis so that appropriate and flexible help can be given to those in genuine need' (ibid.). In the place of payments in the form of grants the Social Fund introduced payments that would for the most part consist of loans, to be paid back by claimants in the form of weekly deductions from their existing benefit.

For the poorest of claimants, whom it is meant to help, the Social Fund operates like a nightmare from Alice in Wonderland. Since the amount of money it is able to distribute is strictly limited, and this in turn is allocated to local offices,

> there is such wide – and unexplained – variation in success rates for applications to different Department of Social Security offices (and within the same office to different Social Fund officers) that the chances of a successful application often resemble a lottery.
>
> (Becker and Craig 1989: 14)

As one Social Fund officer recounted, following the introduction of a management-devised matrix prioritising claimants' circumstances in numbered boxes ranging from 1 to 33, 'In some weeks we pay for numbers one to nine, in others one to fifteen, depending on the budget. The use of priorities and circumstances varies from week to week, from office to office' (cited Craig 1988: 16). In an even more surreal twist, the chances of success depend not only on meeting the priority criteria in the right office at the right time, but also on the claimant's ability to repay the loan. By 1996 more than half a million claimants had been refused a loan because it was considered they were too poor to pay back to the government what they would owe (Craig 1998: 53).

For the poorest dependent on Income Support the whittling away of entitlements and the decline in the relative value of benefits has matched their growing numbers. Various reports have highlighted the inadequate level of the state's 'safety net' benefit: a safety net from which significant numbers, for example of young people, have been deliberately excluded. One such report, published by the Child Poverty Action Group, calculated that a family of four on Income Support fell £34 a week short of what was required to maintain a basic living – one that included no outings, one return bus fare a week, and an annual day trip to the seaside (*Guardian* 5 November 1993). Another, undertaken by the Food Commission, found that the allowance for the feeding of children under Income Support benefit rates would not even provide the cost of the workhouse diet prescribed for children in 1876 (*Guardian* 1 February 1994). But while all the poor have suffered a fall in their relative standard of living, certain groups have been singled out for particular attention.

## Young people

As a particular target of state concern and activity, the young unemployed have suffered even further cuts and humiliation. Concern for the socialisation in particular of young working-class men into the adult worlds of work and responsibility has long been a preoccupation of the state. For the most part this process of transition is something that has been achieved through the gradual disciplining of the young themselves in the workplace and through the demands of forming and raising a family. From the 1970s, however, signs appeared that this process was breaking down. Youth unemployment rose as employers switched their preferences to married women as a source of relatively cheap labour, and the disciplinary role of the state was called upon to replace the shrinking effect of the market. Partly also as a consequence of the restricted economic opportunities for young people, the age at which couples began to form families began to rise.

The response of government has been to use the social-security system to postpone the achievement of adult status for those dependent on benefits, and to exert increasing pressure, in particular on the youngest, either to enter the low-wage labour market, to enrol in a succession of dubious 'training' schemes or, probably the least affordable to most, to continue in full-time education. It is a policy that has resulted in extending the dependency of young people on their families or, where family support is non-existent, in adding to the impoverishment and misery facing many working-class youths. A survey of 16–26-year-olds estranged from their families conducted by the National Children's Home in 1993 revealed disproportionate levels of physical and mental ill-health. Living on an average of £34 each per week, nearly all had inadequate diets, two-thirds were in debt, and half had considered resorting to shoplifting and theft to survive. According to the National Children's Home's chief executive, 'the years between childhood and adulthood are supposedly the happiest years of your life. In stark contrast these teenagers are trapped in a lifestyle of poverty and despair' (cited *Independent* 9 November 1993).

Since the late 1970s unemployment has had a disproportionate impact on the young and has been particularly concentrated amongst the least qualified and (despite their qualifications) amongst ethnic minorities. Thus a recent Labour Force Survey estimates that 62 per cent of black young men in London aged 16–24 were unemployed – three times the rate for white young men – while the youth unemployment rate in inner-city Manchester, Liverpool and London is six times higher than in mid-Sussex (*Independent* 20 November 1995).

Official unemployment statistics, which count only those unemployed who claim benefit, has, since they were barred from receiving benefit in 1988, excluded most 16- and 17-year-olds. Yet the Labour Force survey shows that one in five of this age group were in neither education or training or employment. Amongst 18–24-year-olds, despite a fall of 11 per cent between 1990 and 1994 in the number of young people as a whole, and a rise in the numbers staying on in education, unemployment rose by a third to over 615,000, while the rate doubled from 9 to 18 per cent (Unemployment Unit 1995). At the beginning of 1996 the unemployment rate for 18- and 19-year-olds was twice as high as the national average, and over 50 per cent higher for 20–24-year-olds (Department of Employment 1996). Over the period from 1990 to 1994 the proportion of young people unemployed for twelve months or more increased from 16 to 24 per cent (Unemployment Unit 1994). By 1996 it was still at this level: out of over half a million unemployed 19–24-year-olds, 136,000 had been out of work for between six and twelve months and 130,000 for over a year (Department of Employment 1996). For those unemployed, and especially for those unemployed for long periods of time, changes made to the state benefit system for young people have had a particularly severe effect.

The depression of young people's expectations – and especially the expectations of young working-class people – that has been a hallmark, even a target, of government policy since 1979 formed the framework for changes in the benefit system for young people. These changes were unrelenting and peculiarly vicious. As Phillips (1989) noted, the changes started during the summer of 1980 when the government determined that school leavers without work could not sign on for benefits in June but had to wait until September. There then followed a further series of changes between 1983 and 1986 that saw first 16- and 17-year-olds, then 18–20 and ultimately all 21–24-year-olds living at home or in lodgings losing their entitlements to rent additions. Parents were affected at the same time if they were on benefit for it was assumed that they would be receiving £10 a week in rent from a working 18-year-old still living at home. And on it went. The government proceeded with tabloid-press assistance to raise the spectre of young unemployed people moving to seaside resorts and living the high life at taxpayers' expense. This resulted in new residence restrictions being imposed with respect to board and lodgings regulations which affected some 85,000 young people, forcing them to move periodically from place to place in order to qualify. By 1987 there had been fourteen cuts in social security that had removed £200 million worth of benefits from young people (Andrews and Jacobs 1990: 77). Then, as Phillips details,

April 1988 brought the introduction of the 1986 Social Security Act which introduced income support, the social fund and family credit. It is easy to forget the scale and importance of those changes, particularly the compound reductions faced by some young people . . . the loss of householder status which used to mean that anyone having to meet their own housing costs received the same help regardless of their age . . . everyone having to pay at least 20% of domestic rates and all their water rates . . . the loss of emergency payments – no money to get a bed for the night . . . .the end of single payments – no more help with deposits for accommodation . . . a 16 or 17 year old with a child on £40 a week compared with an 18 year old on £54 . . . the freezing of child benefit . . . guidelines for the social fund that defined young people as 'better able to cope with a crisis' and made them low priority for cash-limited funds.

(Phillips 1989: 22)

Two changes introduced in 1988 were of particular importance for the young: the first was the disbarring of all but a tightly prescribed group of vulnerable 16- and 17-year-olds from claiming Income Support. The second was the introduction of a lower rate of benefit for all single claimants under the age of 25. Since then 16- and 17-year-olds unable to find a job or a place on a training scheme, without families or with families that are unable or unwilling to support them, have formed a growing number of the destitute and homeless. In 1994 97,000 16–17-year-olds had no work and no training place, and of these only 28,000 received any income, mostly in the form of the tightly controlled Severe Hardship Allowance, which is payable only to those who are at serious risk of abuse or of significant harm to their health (Unemployment Unit 1994). One survey conducted by the Coalition on Young People and Social Security in the early 1990s of young people who had claimed this allowance found that 45 per cent had been or still were homeless, half had no money, a quarter said that they had had to beg, steal or sell drugs in order to survive, a quarter already had criminal convictions, and a quarter of the girls were pregnant (cited Wilkinson 1994: 36).

Although Andrews and Jacobs argue that 'it is hard to escape the conclusion that the young have been deliberately selected as easy targets in the assault against benefits' (Andrews and Jacobs 1990: 74) it is clear that this has not been the only consideration. As the *Times* noted in 1983, the targeting of young people's benefits, while

primarily to allow the DHSS to offer a meaty sacrifice on the altar of the Public Expenditure Survey Committee . . . [is] also, more important for the long run, to establish the violability of basic social benefits and do it for a group over which the political screams will not be too loud.

(cited Allbeson 1985: 86)

Since then basic social benefits once considered inviolable, not only for the young but also for the rest of the poor, have been subject to increasing cut-back and restrictions.

Within a trajectory of increasing inequality the fate of young people is especially significant. As the future generation of adults, parents and workers their experience is crucial in determining what in the future will or will not be considered as acceptable, or at least as unchallengeable. The assault on young people has involved the imposition of new work disciplines, lower expectations in terms of both social-security benefits and job security, pay and conditions, and a sexual, social and moral agenda that the neo-liberal project has pursued in the face of both uncertain evidence and immense hardship to some of the most vulnerable of the young.

## The unemployed

The unemployed, and not only the young but also the long-term unemployed, have been made a particular target. In 1980 the newly elected Conservative government introduced its first Social Security Acts, reducing Unemployment Benefit by 5 per cent, abolishing the earnings-related supplement first introduced in 1966, and, as with all other benefits, ending its automatic link to rising standards of living. In 1984 additional payments for dependent children of the unemployed were abolished, and in 1986 the three-quarter and half rates of benefit payable to those who only partially fulfilled the contribution requirements were ended. By 1994 the value of Unemployment Benefit for a single person was a mere 13 per cent of average earnings (Oppenheim and Harker 1996: 51). It was then that the government announced its intention to replace all existing benefits for the unemployed with a new Jobseeker's Allowance.

The Jobseeker's Allowance, introduced in 1996, replaced both Unemployment Benefit and means-tested Income Support for the unemployed with a common level of benefit set at the lower rate of Income Support payments. Although the difference in the level of the two benefits had never been great, Unemployment Benefit had, since its introduction in 1911, been payable as a matter of right, and regardless of other household income, to those who qualified by virtue of having paid a sufficient number of National Insurance contributions. In 1961 72 per cent of unemployed claimants qualified for Unemployment Benefit, although in the buoyant conditions of the labour market of the time few needed to claim it for long, and even fewer for the twelve months maximum that was allowed. By the 1990s, however, with dramatic changes in the labour market bringing not only long-term unemployment but also increased insecurity of work, and hence the inability of many workers to build up a sufficient contribution record, the number of unemployed claimants who qualified had fallen to 19 per cent. With the introduction of the Jobseeker's Allowance, these workers found their entitlement to the 'contributory allowance' reduced from twelve months to six, after which time they, like the majority of the unemployed, remained eligible for benefit only on the means-tested conditions attached to the non-contributory allowance.

The Jobseeker's Allowance was, however, more than just a move to end what the government's White Paper saw as 'the current two benefits system of support [that] has now outlived its usefulness' (cited Finn and Murray 1995: 304). For both insured and uninsured claimants it also imposed new conditions and restrictions on claimants, hailed by the Conservative Research Department as a series of 'sanctions on the work-shy' (cited *Guardian* 17 January 1996).

According to the White Paper that preceded the introduction of the Jobseeker's Allowance, 'there is still a common misunderstanding that people qualify for benefit by virtue only of being unemployed, and not by what they are doing to find work' (cited Finn and Murray 1995: 304). It is this requirement to demonstrate the effort to find work as a condition of receiving benefit that forms the backbone of both Contributory and Non-Contributory Jobseeker's Allowance alike. Under the Act all unemployed claimants are required to sign a detailed Jobseeker's Agreement. In addition to the requirement for claimants to specify in detail their availability for work, and at what kind of jobs and levels of pay, they now also have to indicate the number of employers they will write to, telephone and visit every week; the number of times they will visit the Jobcentre, the newspapers they will consult for vacancies and the employment agencies they will register with. Failure to agree and sign this Agreement – or subsequently to meet its goals – will result in a suspension from benefit.

In further pursuit of this objective, the Act has also introduced a new mechanism 'at the core of the new tough regime that the unemployed will encounter' (Finn and Murray 1995: 310). The Jobseeker's Directive will according to the White Paper allow officials (in that same newspeak that has turned the unemployed into jobseekers, now called, with no sense of irony, 'client advisers') 'to direct jobseekers to improve their employability through, for example, attending a course to improve job-seeking skills or motivation, or taking steps to present themselves acceptably to employers' (cited Finn and Murray 1995: 311). These unprecedented powers given to client advisers to direct the behaviour, and even the appearance, of claimants greatly increases the scope for discrimination and the operation of personal prejudice, and it is not difficult to imagine which people officials may consider, through their behaviour or appearance, as not making themselves 'acceptable' to employers.

Although the Labour Party in opposition had earlier condemned proposals for the introduction of the Jobseeker's Act, with Gordon Brown, the future Chancellor of the Exchequer, dismissing the proposals as 'more insidious and more threatening than the previous Thatcher reviews' and arguing that they went 'right to the heart of the welfare state' (*Independent* 22 November 1993), signs were now to emerge that New Labour's leadership had something other than wholesale abolition in mind should they come to power. In May 1996 Brown was reported to have vetoed a proposal to restore the six-month contributory benefit to twelve months. At the same time, Michael Meacher, the Labour Party's employment spokesman, was required by the Labour leadership to retract a claim that 'the Jobseeker's Allowance is unacceptable and Labour will abolish it' (*Telegraph* 20 May 1996). According to the employment editor of the *Financial Times*, 'the Labour leader is keen to avoid any charge from the Conservatives that his party would be soft on welfare recipients' (*Financial Times* 10 July 1996).

'There is', argued Sir Ralph Howell, Conservative MP for Norfolk North, during the Bill's second reading, 'something awful about insisting people should go on writing application letters when there was no work available . . . It's like forcing people to play bagatelle on a board which has no holes in it' (cited *Guardian* 11 January 1995). Ever since the 1832 Poor Law Commission noted the widespread use of practices 'to force the applicants to give up a certain portion of their time by confining them in a gravel pit or some other enclosure, or directing them to sit at a certain spot and do nothing, or obliging them to attend a roll-call several times a day, or by any contrivance which shall prevent their leisure from becoming a means either of profit or of amusement' (Checkland and Checkland (eds) 1974: 89) the state has taken a perverse delight in what one former social-security official described as 'mucking claimants about'.

Although, as the experience of many claimants testifies, this is a constant and enduring feature of the social-security system, its history also reveals that such pressures are increased at times of greatest poverty and need. It was the first 'great depression' of the 1880s and 1890s that saw a concerted 'Campaign Against Outdoor Relief' directed by the Poor Law authorities against the able-bodied unemployed (Novak 1988: 93–5), while the Not Genuinely Seeking Work Test introduced into the 1927 Unemployed Insurance Act was to force hundreds of thousands of unemployed to tramp from workplace to workplace during the inter-war years in order to demonstrate their search for work. The third great depression of the 1980s and 1990s has similarly seen an escalating series of measures that put barriers in the way of claimants, supposedly to test their willingness and availability for work while for millions there is simply no work available. Such pointless tasks, experienced more often as a punishment than an aid in finding work, can scarcely be seen, in the words of Michael Portillo, as 'designed to improve work incentives' (*Guardian* 22 November 1995), except to the extent to which they so alienate claimants that they take whatever work is available, no matter how much poorer they become.

This eventuality is of course also part of the agenda. As Lord Inglewood, minister in the House of Lords, revealed when rejecting an amendment that would protect claimants from having to take work that paid less than the state's minimum benefit allowance, 'we believe people should not hold out indefinitely for a given level of remuneration . . . After six months we would expect the jobseeker to place no restriction on the rate of pay' (*Independent* 17 May 1995).

The increase in the number of low-paid workers, and the widening inequalities of wages amongst those in work, testify to the pressures that the unemployed face to take whatever work is available. Yet even in these conditions there are limits to the extent to which the economy is capable of absorbing many of the unemployed, even at the lowest rates of pay. This is particularly true for unskilled workers, whose opportunities for employment have fallen markedly. With declining employment prospects for the unskilled, for black people and for working-class youth, who figure disproportionately amongst the unemployed, the measures introduced by the Jobseeker's Allowance serve only as a form of punishment.

Whereas previously suspending a claimant from benefit required the decision of an independent adjudication officer, the decision to suspend benefit for two weeks (rising to four if the offence is repeated) for not being available for or not actively seeking work, for failing to complete a Jobseeker's Agreement or follow a Jobseeker's Directive, including attending a training scheme or employment programme, are now to be made by client advisers. During this time, only those claimants with children, who are pregnant, sick or disabled or with caring responsibilities will be able to claim a reduced hardship payment – and then only if they can prove that they are 'suffering hardship' – other claimants will not receive benefit, or even access to the Social Fund. Similarly, those claimants deemed to have left their previous job 'voluntarily' continue to be subject to a maximum of twenty-six weeks' disqualification, but unlike previously are no longer automatically eligible to claim hardship payments.

Many of these sanctions have existed for many years. More have been introduced since the 1980s, and all have been applied with increasing severity, especially since the introduction in 1994 of performance targets for Employment Service staff which specified targets for suspension and disqualification. Since then the application of sanctions has increased three-fold, with almost a third of a million claimants suspended for not actively seeking work or not attending 'remotivation' courses (Unemployment Unit Press Release 1 August 1996). The Jobseeker's Allowance, however, is likely substantially to increase these sanctions further in line with its increased powers, while the consequences for claimants will be considerably more severe.

## A rock and a hard place

> But of course deprivation is getting worse. I sit in my surgery every week in Chesterfield and whereas when I was elected it was a matter of clearing up a few little bureaucratic hiccups in the welfare state, now people come and burst into tears; they can't manage, they can't live on the money, they're homeless, they're single parent mums. It's like being a stretcher bearer at the bloody battle of the Somme.
>
> (Tony Benn interview in *New Internationalist* July 1996: 25)

For many people, the closing decades of the twentieth century have seen their world turned upside down. What were once certainties in their lives have crumbled to dust before their eyes. Their aspirations about their own neighbourhoods, their workplaces, a notion that governments had some sort of responsibility to ensure that they didn't end up in destitution on the streets, the idea that their own children would do at least as well as themselves, have all been shaken and disturbed. Even old verities such as the security of bricks and mortar were proved false for thousands of people when the value of their newly acquired homes crashed. For those with the least in Britain it has been, as Tony Benn described, like the bloody battle of the Somme. And again the 'generals' prosper in the midst of slaughter.

The combined effect of the deterioration of the labour market and the onslaught on state benefits has been, to continue with the war analogy, like a co-ordinated pincer movement with incredible pressure applied on those caught between. For those with the least skills, social and economic power it has been a classic lose–lose scenario, squeezed by unemployment, low pay and casualisation on the one hand, and an increasingly parsimonious and brutalising social-security system on the other. For successive Conservative governments since 1979, and now it would seem the New Labour administration, this onslaught has been necessary for working people to come to terms with the new realities of an anti-social and global capitalism. Consequently, the rhetoric (and some of the practice) of the social-democratic welfare state has been stripped away. Led by Britain and the USA, a new common sense has argued that these old welfare settlements were literally demoralising working people, especially those most vulnerable and exposed to the new economic realities of triumphal global capitalism. If they were to avoid a future of impoverishment and join the winners, it was their duty to become more flexible, to get on their bikes in search of new opportunities, to get trained, not to be bothered about wages, or health and safety, for once in work the job escalator would take them upwards. This was what global capitalism demanded if the old centres were to compete with the new realities of mobile transnational corporations which in their pursuit of profit would move to those regions and countries which did not burden them with what they considered as unreasonable costs or political demands with respect to workers' rights and rewards.

There is no longer much sense that the welfare state is there to help in periods of crisis, or that governments through macro-economic management will seek to intervene to create new employment opportunities. On the contrary, the welfare state has through a torrent of measures been fundamentally recast and its 'caring' functions have been increasingly superseded by its regulatory and surveillance functions. The consequences for both the workers and users of the welfare system have been bewildering as they have been bombarded by legislation in a context of unrelenting cuts, year on year. It would be possible to fill this book with similar examples from nurses, doctors, probation officers, lecturers in higher and further education, indeed any user or worker in the public sector. The transfer of billions of pounds from social spending (Davies 1997: 293 estimated that Margaret Thatcher had stripped out

£12 billion by 1987) is evident everywhere in the literally crumbling infrastructure of so many public institutions, especially those which are most used by poor people. Visit any town and city and it is difficult to avoid the sight of closed and boarded-up community centres, youth clubs and doctors' surgeries, Victorian school and hospital buildings with leaking roofs, drab paintwork and the rest. The eyes alone confirm what has been occurring over the past two decades – the degradation of the social which we discuss in further detail later in the book.

But in terms of impoverishment, this transformation of the social-democratic welfare state created after the second world war is like a further twist of the knife. As the changes in the labour market and social-security systems remove material certainties and securities and significantly add to the pressures and tensions of poverty so the very services one might need in such circumstances evaporate before your eyes. Instead, hard-pressed families and households are told that it is not the responsibility of the state to intervene, but rather their responsibility – and that they will feel all the better for doing so. Hardly any wonder that late twentieth-century Britain is taking on ever more characteristics of an earlier century with charities being overwhelmed by demand as the state retreats and abandons the poor.

# 3 The abuse of the poor

> An inescapable truth of human and other higher mammalian relationships is that those who are respectfully treated are likely to be respectful to others.
>
> (Kraemer and Roberts 1996: 5)

It is not difficult to find evidence that the poor are generally held to be unworthy of respect. The language and terms used may have changed in some respects over time, but the sense of condemnation and disrespect remains constant. The sense of their expendability as worthless citizens is never far from the surface. Take for example the following exchange in one of the enquiries into deaths in police custody:

MR KILROY-SILK: Dr Johnson, you are the man who sees the result of deaths in police custody. Do you think that there is any real justifiable concern about the number of deaths in police custody?

DR JOHNSON: No I do not, frankly. The people who die in police custody are, for the most part, people, if I may say so, at risk; they are alcoholics, drug addicts, people wandering at large, vagrants, the underprivileged, let us call them. I think that they are at risk anyway.

(cited Scraton 1984: 65)

This exchange is brutally clear: poor people do not count. They, like the million people in the third world who die each year as a direct result of poverty, are expendable. When their death comes at the hands of the state and its agents, as with the death squads of Latin America who clear the streets of the homeless and impoverished as if they were garbage, it reflects a construction of its victims as less than human beings, for how else can such violence be sustained? Racism, with its enduring legacy that has described black people as animals, savages and inferior, is a powerful contributor to this. The police officer in Manchester who, in the course of an investigation into policing methods in Moss Side – a predominantly black and poor area of the city – described its residents as 'wall to wall shit' (*Statewatch* 4(6) (1994): 3) expressed a view that is all too common, and which has contributed to the disproportionate number of deaths of black people in police custody.

The abuse of the poor, while extending at one extreme to the taking of their lives occurs across a wide continuum. At the other end is the daily lack of respect afforded to poor people, and in between there is ritual humiliation, emotional, physical and sexual abuse. What is most telling about this is that those who are the greatest victims of poverty and its many consequences – the homeless, the disturbed, the most vulnerable – are frequently the most abused.

## Policing

In his account of the Broadwater Farm disturbances, the investigative journalist David Rose (1992) noted that the then chief of the London police, Kenneth Newman, had argued that one of his force's greatest challenges was the policing of the London ghettos. According to Newman, these were the modern-day rookeries of London, inhabited by people who lived their lives outside the normal rules of society – people so far removed from so-called civilised living that there was no point in trying to enter into any dialogue about the needs and problems of their estates. Instead they were seen as intrinsically opposed to the police – the enemy within. For such people there was no place for the sort of police liaison work advocated by Lord Scarman after the Brixton riots. This particular construction of such poor and deprived neighbourhoods had a decisive impact on the type of policing they received and experienced. As Rose observed:

> Press reports – and there were many other examples – were portraying the estate as something 'other', alien, 'not England', a jungle. As Tim Miles had hinted in his article in the *Mail*, in such a place, the niceties of civil liberties need not apply. The usual rules of criminal investigation might have to be suspended, or as his interviewee put it, 'I don't care what methods are used to bring some law and order back to Broadwater Farm'.
>
> (Rose 1992: 80)

Later in his account, Rose provides numerous examples of what it meant to the people of this estate when 'the niceties of civil liberties need not apply'.

> In numerous cases they began at dawn with the smashing of doors with sledgehammers and the entry of a squad of armed police. One woman described the police entry to her flat: 'They said, "It's your bastard's birthday tomorrow isn't it?" I said, "What do you mean by that?" and they said, "It's your little bastard's birthday, open the door, we've got a warrant for your arrest". When I opened the door the sledgehammer was coming back on the door. They grabbed me, they put me to spread out on the wall, and they searched me. All I had on was my tee shirt and knickers . . . it's not affected me, it's my daughter, because she saw everything that happened and she was screaming, literally screaming when she saw, especially when the gun was at my head, you know, she was really, really screaming.'
>
> (Rose 1992: 110–11)

At the root of this police brutality is the understanding of the poor as being worthless – counting for nothing: an attitude which has a long and terrible history, as reflected in Hannington's account of an episode in the struggles of the Birkenhead Unemployed Workers in 1932:

> The screams of the women and children were terrible, we could hear the thuds of the blows from the batons and the terrific struggles in the rooms below. . . . Presently our door was forced open . . . Twelve police rushed into the room and immediately knocked down my husband, splitting open his head and kicking him as he lay on the floor. The language of the police was terrible. When I tried to prevent them hitting my husband they commenced to baton me all over the arms and body; as they hit my husband and me the children were screaming and the police shouted: 'Shut-up you parish-fed bastards.'
>
> (cited Green 1990: 17)

But this behaviour of the police is not simply confined to moments of high drama such as the Broadwater Farm or Birkenhead Unemployment riots, nor to a few individuals who might be seen as exceptions to the rule. Instead, as with the endemic racism of the police being revealed at the time of writing in the public enquiry into the murder of Stephen Lawrence, there is considerable evidence that the police hold deeply prejudicial views of all those who are the most disadvantaged. In a speech to the 1982 Conservative Party conference, one of the vice chairs of the Police Federation argued that

> In every urban area there is a large minority of people who are not fit for salvage. They hate every form of authority – whether it is the police or anybody else. The only way that the police can protect society is, quite frankly, by harassing these people so that they are afraid to commit crime.
>
> (cited Bridges 1983: 36)

The implications of such an approach were clearly illustrated by Bea Campbell (1993) when she noted how the policing of the most deprived council-house estates is typically informed by a negative stigmatising perception which embraces the entire neighbourhood, and which sees all its residents as useless and rotten. As a consequence a 'normal' police presence and approach was abandoned as being too dangerous. Rather policing was episodic and in strength. Police rarely responded to individual calls for help on the estates and left the community to manage as best it could. But every so often, as tensions mounted, the police would enter as an invading force, tooled up for action with protected vans and helicopter support, and sweep up all those out on the streets irrespective of their behaviour or conduct. To live in such an area designates one as criminal. It is a crushing response. It is also one which enshrines a sense of impunity both with respect to the perpetrators and the victims. This impunity emboldens the abusers (for who is there to speak out against such atrocities?) as much as it undermines the victims, who know that nobody in authority appears to care what it is done to them.

## Counting for nothing

It is not, however, only in the policing of poor people and communities, or in the excesses of powerful individuals, that such abuse takes place. Take a look at the public agencies that predominantly if not exclusively deal with the poor: at the means-tested benefit system and social-services departments, or even the hospitals, doctors' surgeries and schools of the supposedly 'universal' welfare state that are situated in poor areas. It has become a truism within social policy that those services provided by the state which are specifically aimed only at the poor are invariably poor services. A few years ago, a group of students were assigned to visit a range of welfare organisations which dealt with predominantly poor people. Their task was simply to visit and observe, to see if they could determine the agencies' attitudes towards their users on the basis of their observations of the buildings, their layout, the reception areas and the general facilities available. The organisations visited ranged from citizens' advice centres, well-women clinics to the local social-security office, social-services and probation departments. Their findings and responses were illuminating. They talked of the voluntary-sector agencies in generally positive terms; of their bright and welcoming decor, smart and comfortable furniture, of the pot plants, of notice boards with up-to-date information, of toys for children to play with in the reception areas, of signs indicating the location of toilets and of good access for people with disabilities. The state agencies on the other hand were described quite differently: austere and shabby environments, uncomfortable seating, some of it secured to the ground, tatty notice boards, old and dog-eared magazines in the reception areas with no toys for the kids, even toilets where the toilet paper was the cheapest and nastiest available. They gave particular attention in these agencies to the grilles and barriers which divided the staff from the users and the humiliation which resulted as people had to shout out their business and difficulties in front of all those waiting in order to be heard by the officials. Moreover in the state agencies the students were invariably interrogated as to the purpose of their visit and the university was contacted by the manager of the social-security office who wanted to know what was going on, who was responsible and why he had not been warned of the visit to this public institution.

The students' conclusions were as revealing as they were anticipated. The state agencies were seen as hostile places which made you feel 'guilty', 'on edge' and unwelcome. The voluntary agencies on the other hand were generally perceived as welcoming, wanting to set you at ease and concerned to help. These were conclusions based primarily on observation and relatively little discussion with those working in the organisations. The observations echoed those of Becker and Silburn, whose research on the impact of the Social Fund brought them into contact with social-services departments. Social work, once seen as a 'helping' agency, or at least intended to be so, has over the past twenty years been transformed. Such was the impact of this change that they felt compelled in their report to note:

> We have formed a striking impression as we visited local social work area offices that gradually but by now quite unmistakably they are coming to resemble DSS offices. The tackiness of the furniture, the torn magazines, the broken toys, the doors that can only be opened by tapping in a code number, the separation of client

and worker by partitions or glass screens, the increasing use of appointment systems, the air, even the smell, of drab, down-at-heel despair in the waiting rooms, this is now commonly encountered in many places, as though working with the new poor clients creates a poor working environment.

(Becker and Silburn 1990: 81)

The message given by such organisations (even before you engage with the staff) is clear. They are places for losers. Visiting is a deeply corrosive, undermining and ultimately damaging experience and one which for many people is repeated continually over long periods of time. For the very poorest, contact with such agencies as social work, education welfare officers, social security and housing officials is usually the most extensive. People's lives are taken up in endless waiting and queues, in being shunted from office to office as if their time was of no importance. When the reception they receive is indifferent or hostile it compounds a sense of worthlessness and eats away at self-confidence.

Of course when looking at poverty, and especially the experiences of those who are most dependent on state welfare institutions for their income or other resources, it is essential that benefit levels are considered. But if the social relations embedded in these transactions are ignored then a major part of the story is omitted. For it is often in these relationships and interactions that so much of the abuse of the poor takes place.

## More civilised methods

The surplus population has to be kept in ignorance, but also controlled. The problem is faced directly in the Third World domains that have long been dominated by the West and therefore reflect the guiding values of the masters most clearly: here favoured devices include death squads, 'social cleansing', torture and other techniques of proven effectiveness. At home, more civilised methods are (still) required.

(Chomsky 1996: 6)

Social work, which was taken up from its private charitable origins and expanded considerably by the state after the second world war, represents for many people the compassionate and civilised face of welfare. Working with the most impoverished and often the most damaged casualties of poverty, it is seen as an indication of the nation's capacity and willingness to 'care' for its most vulnerable members. The revelations of systematic emotional, physical and sexual abuse that came to light in Britain in the early 1990s, in a succession of official inquiries into the care of children in state institutions, tells a different story. For some of the most vulnerable and abused, being taken into the 'care' of the state was the beginning of a process of yet further and organised abuse from those employed to care for them.

Social work is a challenging profession. Its clients include some of the most generous, warm and compassionate people – qualities that abound amongst the poor – as well as some of the most damaged, disfigured and self-destructive. These two faces of poverty present a considerable challenge to social work: one belies the view of the poor, and especially of the poorest, as barbaric and uncivilised; the other appears to confirm it in full measure. Throughout the history of social work social workers have been confronted with evidence that the people they work with are the casualties of a society that holds them of no regard, while the social-work profession, the training of its recruits and the practices of the agencies which employ them have reinforced the view that the problems clients experience are mainly of their own making.

Social workers deal almost exclusively with the very poorest. When Alvin Schorr, the distinguished American sociologist, was invited to provide an outsider's view of contemporary personal social services in the UK he opened his chapter on clients with the following observation:

> The most striking characteristics that clients of the personal social services have in common are poverty and deprivation. *Often this is not mentioned*, possibly because the social services are said to be based on universalistic principles. Still, everyone in the business knows it. One survey after another shows that clients are unemployed or, to observe a technical distinction, not employed – that is, not working and not seeking work. Perhaps half receive income support, as many as 80 per cent have incomes at or below income support levels.
>
> (Schorr 1992: 8; emphasis added)

Despite their heterogeneity – including older people, those with various forms of disability and long-term illness, young people and households often under severe emotional and financial stress – the clients of social work share many common characteristics. They are from the point of view of capital a surplus population, who either because of age, disability or lack of skills have the most marginal if any relationship to waged labour. They are often geographically concentrated in the poorest and most run-down areas, rarely owning their homes, rarely in paid work, with few if any financial resources. They are the poorest of the poor, containing at their core many of those who over time have been called the undeserving poor, the residuum, problem families and now the underclass.

For many of these social work is the last resort. When housing and social-security officials, the education department and other agencies of the state refuse them help, social work remains as the last 'safety net'. But it is a safety net with many holes, and one that comes at a high price. For many, to call upon the social services – or, more accurately, to be referred to them, since the vast majority of clients do not go willingly but are sent by the courts or other state welfare agencies – is a surrender. It is to expose the intimate details of family, personal, emotional and financial life to a stranger, who expects 'co-operation' and in return may be able to offer help: to twist the arm of social-security officials, to press for rehousing or urgent repairs, or to arrange temporary respite from the pressing stresses that the poor encounter. Money rarely changes hands: social-services departments are severely limited in the financial aid they can give, and in general view clients as untrustworthy and dishonest. Often the best that is on offer is friendly advice; at worst a moral condemnation – backed by extensive powers to remove children from families – which demands changes in values, attitudes and behaviour in return for assistance.

Social work has, since its origins in the 'charitable' efforts of the Charity Organisation Society during the last quarter of the nineteenth century, been deeply ambivalent about the poor. Throughout this history social work itself has not merely reflected dominant attitudes but has also been a crucial agency in the shaping and legitimating of those beliefs. Primary amongst these has been the view that poverty and inequality are not the most significant factors in the reproduction of the client population or of the multiple difficulties many of them encounter. Rather, this view has persisted in maintaining that the poverty and disadvantage of clients is not a result of social factors and systems but a symptom of the clients' inadequacy of character and morality. The monthly journal of the COS stated this clearly:

> There can be no doubt that the poverty of the working classes of England is due, not to their circumstances (which are more favourable than those of any working population of Europe); but to their improvident habits and thriftlessness. If they are ever to be more prosperous, it must be through self-denial, temperance and forethought.
>
> (*Charity Organisation Review* 10 (1881): 50)

Mainstream social-work texts over the past century, when they have bothered to discuss poverty at all, have maintained this fiction, that the poverty of clients is not the 'real issue', but rather a 'presenting problem' behind which 'lies not just a lack of money, or even financial mismanagement, but deeper disturbances in family relationships' (Rodgers 1960: 89). This is exemplified by the social worker who argued that 'it's not a question of poverty but mismanagement or emotional difficulties which make them spend money the wrong way – you can manage [on welfare benefits] but it's not the kind of thing an inadequate person can do' (cited Smith and Harris 1972: 38–9).

This idealistic orientation of social work whereby ideas, values and personal morality are held to be the primary determinants of material and social condition has contributed greatly to the sense that those at the bottom of the social pile are different and defective human beings. Its lack of a materialist perspective, coupled with a general acceptance of the bourgeois values of thrift, independence and sobriety, has left the behaviour of those who fail to live up to these norms inexplicable, except as the result of innate deficiencies or inadequate upbringing. Over the years, social work has plundered the social sciences, especially psychology, to provide legitimation for this perspective. In doing so social work has presented its clients in the most disrespectful manner. According to one influential British social-work leader, a 'great number' of clients 'resemble greedy demanding children, always clamouring for material help, always complaining of unfair treatment or deprivation; this attitude shades into paranoid imagining or provoking of slights and rebuffs' (Irvine 1954: 27). In the double bind that characterises many of the encounters between the state and the poor, those who complain or are resentful, even angry, towards those supposedly there to help them are further pathologised:

> Over and over again one senses, beneath a hostile veneer, an oral character; a client who never stops demanding . . . The dependency is pervasive and the client sucks from neighbours, shopkeepers, bartenders and news vendors as well as family members and social workers.
>
> (cited Richan and Mendelsohn 1973: 15)

It was on such foundations that the state turned to social work and sponsored its development and expansion after 1945. The long capitalist boom of the 1950s and 1960s created a thirst for labour which determined that all available sources of it should be secured for the economy. From the point of view of the state there was little of compassion in this.

Whereas in its earlier 'charitable' form, social work had dismissed 'the residuum' as beyond help or redemption, and had distrusted the impersonal hand of the state as incapable of reforming people's character, now social work was to become a mainstream state activity focused on the poorest of the poor. This significant change of orientation to the most vulnerable and impoverished was not driven principally by humanitarian concerns, although in the immediate post-1945 period there was a popular demand to be rid of the legacy of the cruel Poor Law and the creation of a welfare society which was genuinely more compassionate and concerned. Whilst these attitudes were important, the revolution in the approach to the poorest was principally driven by the economic need to secure the most productive use of all able-bodied people to feed the long boom – investment in human capital as it was commonly termed. The children of problem families in this context were seen as wasted labour who, whilst constituting an estimated 10 per cent of the population (Women's Group on Public Welfare 1943), rarely made it to the labour market in a fit state, becoming instead delinquents, prostitutes, inmates of mental hospitals and expensive, long-term dependants on the recently expanded welfare state.

The promise offered by social work was that it had the tools and knowledge base to intervene amidst the most deprived and damaged communities to rescue and restore especially the children of 'problem families' and to turn them into productive citizens. Informed by the more optimistic insights of psychoanalysis which asserted the possibilities of treatment and rehabilitation as against the earlier pessimism of biological determinism which offered no such prospects, social work made grandiose promises about its capacity to rid society of long-term welfare dependency, the spectre of juvenile delinquency and general unemployability amongst the most impoverished. The key to this promise lay in social casework, whereby social workers would enter into the lives of these so-called dysfunctional families and through a personal relationship re-educate and re-moralise the poorest, breaking down the cycle of deprivation and its culture of poverty. Social casework would decrease the need for expensive institutions, reduce welfare dependency and above all bring into use labour power that would otherwise have been unavailable.

As long as the boom continued, the state hesitatingly sponsored the expansion and development of social work. Especially with regard to work with children and their families it epitomised the social-democratic welfare state. The very fact that the poorest were now considered as suitable for rehabilitation rather than simple control and containment gave social work a liberal and compassionate reputation. Quite unlike any other previous form of state intervention in its personalised style and gentle approach, it depended on a trusting relationship between the social worker and the client as a precondition of the internal changes in attitudes and values which were held to be the goals of social work's intervention. Such change, social work insisted, could not be brought about through shouting and imposed regulation but demanded a more empathic stance.

The state's development and sponsorship of social work throughout the era of social democracy was, however, always contested. The conjuncture of psychoanalytical ideas, economic necessity and political will which were so crucial to social work's expansion did not sweep away deeply sedimented ideas about its clients. There were similarly held views within other sections of the state, especially the police and the judiciary, as well as amongst conservatives, that problem families were not capable of reform and that the softly-softly approach of social work would be abused by them. The idea that problem families were deprived and in need of help was anathema to those who maintained that they were depraved and that an iron fist rather than a velvet glove was all that such families would understand. Such ideas were never vanquished, and as already noted, were to return with a vengeance once the economic imperative of utilising all possible sources of labour evaporated from the mid-1970s onwards.

However, even in its social-democratic form, social work for all its emphasis on developing warm and trusting relationships with clients never really challenged the idea that those at the bottom of the social system were to blame for their plight. Indeed, as a result of its close contact and involvement with 'problem families' in particular, it contributed significantly to strengthening the notion that their social position reflected their inadequacies and their failings. Focusing particularly on family dynamics, social work reinforced rather than weakened conceptions of pathologisation in which women as mothers were castigated for their failure to socialise appropriately their (many) children. For all their psycho-social rhetoric, social workers diagnosed the problems presented by clients as being rooted not in their poverty but in their flawed personalities. In many respects their incursions into the underbelly of British society were similar to those of the missionaries of colonial Britain. There was nothing to learn from the 'natives'; social workers were the carriers of the 'truth' and bringers of civilisation.

With the expansion of social work, the tentacles of the state extended ever deeper into the lives of the poorest. Detailed dossiers are compiled, rarely accessible to those whose lives are described and judged, increasingly shared amongst a wide range of state agencies, and which form the basis of social-work activity. The price of social-work 'help' is all too often state supervision. For many, the implications of their contact with social-work agencies can be devastating, especially in such high-profile instances as child abuse. Adele Jones (1993) observed:

> There are many people who have found the effects of social work intervention to be as great as, and sometimes greater than the effects of abuse. 'I asked you [reported one client] to put an end to the abuse – you put an end to my whole family, you took away my nights of hell and gave me days of hell instead; you've exchanged my private nightmare for a very public one'.
>
> (Jones 1993: 78)

For clients, contact with social workers is commonly dominated by their powerlessness which is deepened as social workers come increasingly to be the gateways through which other state resources are accessed. Co-operation and sometimes changes in behaviour are thereby crudely secured by social workers withholding resources. Handler noted how a family had been refused any financial assistance over a period of two months:

> During this time, it was made plain that this lever was being used until more co-operative efforts were forthcoming. The [child care] officer wanted a better work effort from the husband and a change in attitude as to what the family thought was owing to them from the welfare state.
>
> (Handler 1968: 486)

He concluded by noting:

> That the operative principles in the Children's Departments today are remarkably similar to those of the Charity Organisation Society, founded about one hundred years ago. The close supervision of the spending of money is little different from the old system of relief in kind; poor people cannot be trusted to spend money that isn't 'theirs'.
>
> (Handler 1968: 487)

The view of social work from below has been largely negative. There is a widespread sensibility in many working-class neighbourhoods that social workers are to be avoided because of their powers to remove children or commit people to mental hospitals. There is very little trust, and as one client noted 'most of them [social workers] are disgusted by us' and another noted how 'all we want is for social workers to come across to us as people' (Eaton 1996: 10). Bryan and her co-authors in their book on the experiences of black women's lives in Britain provide a graphic sense of their hostility to social work:

> Whether we are single parents, homeless young women or the parents of children in care, we are constantly confronted with racist, classist or culturally biased judgements about our lives. The social background of most social workers and the training they receive give them no real understanding of our different family structures, cultural values and codes of behaviour. It is so much easier for them to rely on loose assumptions and loaded stereotypes of us than to try seriously to address the root cause of our problems. These assumptions become the justification for everything from secret files and surveillance to direct intervention of the most destructive kind.
>
> (Bryan et al. 1985: 112)

Black people have, with good reason, been amongst the most trenchant critics of social work and have accused it of robbing their families of children and placing them in highly inappropriate and abusive children's homes or foster care. They have accused social workers of having little understanding of matriarchal family care in the case of black families coming from the Caribbean. As a consequence of social work's reification of the two-parent family model, any deviation from this norm is regarded as deficient and flawed. This in turn has led to disproportionate numbers of young black offenders being given custodial sentences and removed into care because their household composition is not regarded as a suitable environment for a non-custodial sentence. Informed until the late 1980s by a determined colour-blind approach where the impact of 'race' and racism was ignored, black children were commonly denied their racial identity and suffered appalling personal damage as they struggled to make sense of racism:

> A young person from the Manchester Black and In Care Group describes the way in which she was affected by this process: 'The image of myself was reflected back as an image associated with drugs, violence, simpleness, exotic, problematic, bad and mad. From the time I first saw or heard, all the positive images I was

provided with were white people and I did not exist as myself, or only in someone else's design.'

(Jones 1993: 84)

In an NSPCC report on runaway children, one similarly gains a sense of social workers being seen as part of the problem and not the solution, for the young people concerned. According to Barter:

the young people in this study identified that they generally did not feel listened to by their social workers. Neither did they feel respected or consulted about the decisions made about them, nor did they feel that there had been any negotiation in relation to choice of placements. All of the young people now rated their relationships with their social workers as poor.

(Barter 1996: 40)

Here are some of the comments made by the young people about their social workers:

I asked them [social workers] not to see me because every time they came they would wind me up . . . All they ever done was rap, rap, rap. Not a word could I ever get in. He didn't want to know what my views were about the place . . . I was just sitting there listening, listening and listening.

My social worker wanted me to fill these forms in [to make the foster placement permanent]. I'm saying that I'm not happy there and I just want to be moved to another foster home in London . . . He had the cheek to come forward with some forms and ask me if I wanted to make it a permanent thing. Me staying there? After all I'd said. Then he said he'd leave the forms in case I changed my mind . . . He's a real dope.

I knew she [the social worker] was not listening. She was just looking at something while I was speaking. It made me feel worse; made me feel like nobody wanted to listen to me . . . I just expect it now . . . I don't ever want to see her because she makes me feel miserable.

(all cited Barter 1996: 40)

Not hearing the anguish of the poor and vulnerable is one of the key characteristics of their abuse. It is one of the clearest of all indicators of disrespect – that they count for nothing. Although there are very few studies of clients, when their voices are heard this fundamental disrespect is all too evident, with clients both young and old commonly making reference to the fact that they didn't count – 'I suppose they [social workers] thought I was just no good and not worth bothering with' (A. Thompson 1996: 14) being an all too typical comment. Such a perspective contributes significantly to their continued abuse, unless, like the young people in the NSPCC report, they run away – and even then it is too often from one set of abuses to another, as so vividly portrayed by Nick Davies (1997).

The recent spate of enquiries into sustained and large-scale physical and sexual abuse of young people in state residential institutions vividly illustrates the extreme consequences of this situation. For many of the children and young people concerned their removal from their families to these institutions was on the grounds of neglect and sometimes abusive home lives. What they came to encounter was nothing less than torture. In his coverage of one of the enquiries, Nick Davies reported:

> One witness after another describes how they grew up in a world of threats. 'We were treated like animals, creatures, rubbish, . . . there was a fear that one day perhaps someone was going to kill you and perhaps this time it would be done.'
>
> (*Guardian* 24 September 1997)

Davies continued:

> Without power to resist, the children were utterly vulnerable to the paedophiles who had infiltrated the homes. They became sex objects – in the dormitory, and in the sick bay – . . . in the showers, in the staff room, in the bath, in cars, in sheds, in tents, on the towpath of the canal; with men, with women, with residential workers, social workers, and with anyone else who wanted them. . . .
>
> The paedophiles became quite casual. [One] would line boys up in the corridor outside his room and pick a weak one for his entertainment. One careworker is said to have wandered into the dormitory one or two nights a week, like someone in a supermarket. He would choose a boy, call out his name and take him away.
>
> (*Guardian* 24 September 1997)

Moreover, as this and other enquiries have revealed, the young people and children often complained. Some would attempt to escape only to be returned to their place of torture by their social workers, who refused to listen. Some took their own lives; others tried but failed, only to succeed later as adults. They tried to make priests, police officers and other social workers listen. But to no avail. In North Wales the police were formally asked to investigate on twenty-seven occasions and in each case their 'inquiries came to nothing':

> One boy, who described a particularly long and vivid catalogue of abuse said he grabbed hold of the jacket of an executive from social services . . . who was visiting the home. He pleaded with him to do something. 'He just wouldn't listen. He wasn't having any of it.'
>
> (*Guardian* 24 September 1997)

Incredibly, some within the British Association of Social Workers have argued that social workers are listening but do nothing because of resource constraints; the lack of residential provision means that it can be difficult to move clients (Thompson 1996: 14).

The social-work occupation in particular, and governments more generally, would like people to believe that such torture is not wide-spread and is restricted to a small number of 'bad apples' who manage to slip through selection and recruitment systems: that it is a problem that can be solved by technical fixes such as establishing a general social-care council that will regulate more closely the activities of its accredited members. The response is not dissimilar to social workers' attitudes to the revelations of sexual abuse in many families during the latter part of the 1980s in north-east England: it was not a matter of patriarchy and male violence, but again a few bad fathers. What those in power cannot tolerate is that abuse on the scale revealed in some children's homes – and it is highly probable in all institutional settings which supposedly care for the vulnerable poor – flows from the systemic disregard which derives from a conception of sections of the population as being worthless. This worthlessness feeds into their powerlessness which in turn provides those in power with a sense of impunity in their behaviour. Moreover, it is a process which is self-reinforcing and with many victims, as Scheper-Hughes highlights in her discussion of insti-tutionalised life in an American nursing home for older people:

> The personal names of residents are dropped and they are often addressed as 'you'. Little or no account is taken of expressed wishes so that sooner or later any requests or expressions of personal pref-erence   . . . are extinguished. Passivity sets in. When the body is rolled from one side or the other for perfunctory cleaning, when the body is wheeled conveniently into a corner so that the floor can be more easily mopped, when cleaning staff do little to suppress expressions of disgust at urine, faeces or phlegm out of place – on

clothing, under the nails, on wheelchairs or in wastepaper baskets –
the person trapped inside the failing body may also come to see
themselves as 'dirty', 'vile', 'disgusting', an object or a non-
person . . . Meanwhile, the institutional violence and indifference
are masked as the resident's own state of mental confusion and
incompetence. And everything in the nature of the institution
invites the resident to further regression, to give up, to lose, to
accept his or her inevitable and less than human depersonalised
status.

(Scheper-Hughes 1997: 21–2)

Worthless people are housed in worthless conditions, cared for by staff
who are often poorly paid and trained to manage some of the more difficult and challenging individuals in society. Virtually everything in the
situation reinforces the sense of rejection and sustains an environment
which nurtures violence (see Wardhaugh and Wilding (1993) for a
useful discussion of the corruption of care). Until these issues are confronted the abuse will continue.

The abuse of young people, older people, those with learning disabilities and any other group drawn from the poorest of the population
may be at one end of the continuum of violence. But it overshadows all
those who are continually denied their humanity. It is reflected in the 62
per cent of social workers, interviewed in one research project, who
considered that 'an understanding of the suffering and impoverishment
of various client groups was unimportant' (Bell and Webb 1992: 40). It
is reflected in the countless interactions clients have in the course of
their often extensive entanglement with the state, ranging from housing
authorities to nurseries, schools, doctors, the prison service, probation
officers, social security and social workers. In most of these interactions
they are dealt with as problems, as 'grit in the machine', a nuisance
demanding far too much time and attention. They rarely receive any
positive endorsement in these interactions – there is little praise for
their effort, or their capacity to manage in the most difficult of circumstances. There is virtually no acknowledgement of the damage inflicted
by dominant media messages which portray them as layabouts or
cheats; no understanding that each day can bring further humiliation
and that the daily grind of living in poverty brings frustration, anger
and irritability. In her modest research into the implications of the
Labour government's new deal proposals for lone parents, Haughey
(1998) found that most of the lone parents had been undermined by the
unrelenting negative stereotyping of them in the tabloid press: 'The
media describe us as being scroungers, lazy buggers who don't want to

work and live off the state. This just isn't true, but it means I don't have very high self-esteem' (Trudy, cited Haughey 1998: 47).

These are amongst the feelings which Richard Wilkinson demonstrates in his path-breaking work on how the social relations of inequality and poverty destroy lives and do the most damage:

> From the point of view of the experience of the people involved, if health is being damaged as a result of psychosocial pressures, this matters much more than it would if the damage resulted from the immediate effects of damp housing or poor quality diets. If it were not for the psychosocial effects we are talking about, it would be possible to eat a diet with too many chips and too much fried food and be perfectly happy. The same would be true of smoking and taking too little exercise . . . If these were the major causes of health inequalities and income distribution, then it would not be so far from the truth to say that life for the relatively poor might be shorter, but perhaps not much less sweet, than it was for the rich. But this problem is important because that is so far from the truth. To feel depressed, cheated, bitter, desperate and vulnerable, frightened, angry, worried about debts or job and housing insecurity; to feel devalued, useless, helpless, uncared for, hopeless, isolated, anxious and a failure; these feelings can dominate people's whole experience of life, colouring their experience of everything else. It is the chronic stress arising from feelings like these which does the damage. It is the social feelings which matter, not exposure to a supposedly toxic material environment. The material environment is merely the indelible mark and constant reminder of the oppressive fact of one's failure, of the atrophy of any sense of having a place in a community, and of one's social exclusion and devaluation as a human being.
>
> (Wilkinson 1996: 214–15)

This is where we must start if we are truly concerned to understand the plight of clients – not with some spurious rag-bag of half-digested social-science theories and perspectives which insist on locating the difficulties of clients, their often stressed and fractious relationships, in some malfunctioning of early socialisation processes – usually blaming mothers for failing to raise their children appropriately, or in the case of single-parent families because they have deprived their children of a father. As Wilkinson demonstrates, the social violence of poverty is not in the context of societies such as Britain simply due to a lack of basic material resources. Rather it lies in the values which accompany gross inequalities and social polarisation and the acute stress which follows from a sense of worthlessness and failure. It is in these areas that the damage is done, which corrodes the well-being of households, demoralises and undermines and is largely responsible for the differential mortality rates and health inequalities which remain so prevalent and deep-rooted in contemporary Britain (Smith 1987: ch. 1). As Coates and Silburn noted:

> It is these emotional and moral consequences of being poor that are the hardest to grasp for those who have never experienced such deprivations themselves, but they are at the very heart and substance of poverty. They rob a man [sic] of his pride and his dignity; ultimately they dehumanise him.
>
> (Coates and Silburn 1970: 75)

## Abusive social security

Not surprisingly, many of the attitudes and values which inform social-work practice are also prevalent within the social-security system, and especially within the system of means-tested benefits on which the poorest, by definition, most depend. These two major state agencies which impact most directly on the lives and well-being of the most vulnerable and dependent members of the population share much in common and in their practices and operation do much to exacerbate the experience of poverty.

The growing immiseration of the poor at the hands of the social-security system is itself a form of abuse. But, as always, it is not only the financial consequences of such changes which define the experience of poverty. It is also the social relationships which such changes bring about, and in particular the relationships between claimants and those officials on whom they depend for their income. The nature of this relationship has always been difficult. No matter how sympathetic the official, the power to take decisions that will affect whether someone has enough, or less than enough, to live on places officers in an extremely powerful position in relationship to claimants, and no matter what the rights and entitlements of claimants, such powers are frequently abused. This is especially the case when those who administer the system, as historically has always been the case, are themselves low-paid. It is even more so when official pronouncements and the general culture brands those claiming or receiving benefit as undeserving, as potential cheats and scroungers. Added to this powerful mix has been the effect of an increasing workload for social-security staff on the one hand, in terms both of the numbers of claimants they have to deal with and the increasing complexity of the system, and the increasing restrictions, the declining value of benefits, and the growing poverty and desperation facing claimants on the other.

Some of the consequences of this were brought out in a study conducted in a social-security office in Northern Ireland in the early 1980s. As the author of the study noted, there was a huge disparity between the official policy of the department and the actual reality of dealing with claimants. On the one hand:

> internal memos state that officers must give courteous and prompt attention to all claimants, be patient and attentive in listening to requests, be prompt in replying to correspondence, avoid jargon, give proper consideration to exceptional circumstances and needs, provide an explanation to every claimant of the scheme and of his right and obligations within it, and give proper attention to special circumstances which might affect payment arrangements. Staff are exhorted to adopt these practices 'irrespective of claimants' manner or circumstances' and are told that the 'first consideration for the welfare of claimants is to ensure that they receive their full entitlement'.
>
> (Howe 1985: 51–2)

On the other hand, the simple pressures of work on staff made such goals unattainable:

> The time allotted for interviews is fifteen minutes . . . Interviews are so short that once essential information has been collected and evidence documented, the officer has little, if any, time left over to explain the scheme or to enquire into any special circumstances that may exist . . . Overwhelmingly interviews are used to collect information rather than to impart it.
>
> (Howe 1985: 53)

Other studies have revealed similar pressures on staff, with the result that the greater the claimants' needs or the more complicated their circumstances the more they present a problem to over-worked officials. As one executive officer noted:

> It's all right to talk about rights, but let me tell you that when you're faced with our sort of workload, all you're interested in is getting the job dealt with as best you can. It's all about numbers here, not rights.
>
> (cited Cooper 1985: 9)

In such circumstances, claimants who ask questions, who demand explanations, and who even 'appear self-confident' are

> often described as 'aggressive', 'grasping', 'ungrateful', 'shameless', 'greedy' and so on. In contrast, what may be called the 'ideal' claimant is someone who merely answers questions, produces all the required documents, is polite and grateful and who does not mention complicating matters. Such people are described as 'nice', 'easy', 'poor', 'grateful', 'polite' and so on.
>
> (Howe 1985: 61)

That such distinctions between the 'deserving' and the 'undeserving' are drawn, at least in part, on the basis of claimants' attitude and demeanour, rather than evidence of their need is clear, as Howe points out:

> for the simple reason that in many cases such evidence is not available, either because the interviewer makes little attempt to elicit it, or because the claimant does not mention it . . . In sum, the cumulative and systematic effect of all these practices and resource constraints is not one which victimises a particular set of claimants as is, to some extent, intended; on the contrary, it can be argued that, to one degree or another, the majority of claimants are penalised.
>
> (Howe 1985: 68)

In such circumstances it is not surprising that the frustration of claimants has led to growing conflict with staff:

> In the first six months of 1995 Toxteth unemployment benefit office in Liverpool reported more than one attempted assault on officials every week. Nationally between 1989 and 1994 there were 8,000 reported incidents, including over 1,000 actual physical assaults, many more are thought to go unreported. The Employment Service expects more. According to a leaked internal discussion document, proposing the need for security guards, personal alarms, closed circuit television and more training for staff, 'The introduction of the Jobseeker's Allowance will increase the level of risk of actual and attempted assault and verbal abuse in job centres. The introduction of the new incapacity benefit will bring progressively onto registers some people who are likely to have their income reduced by the change and who may have been

out of the job market for some time, and some of whom will be suffering from mental illness.'

(*Guardian* 18 October 1995)

Social-security offices thus come to resemble a battleground between the poor and their custodians. Open-plan offices, introduced in the attempt to reduce the tension felt to be created by the wire meshes and plate-glass screens of older design, are now increasingly equipped with closed-circuit televisions, panic and alarm buttons, and furniture bolted to the floor. The stress on staff working under such conditions is considerable. As one Department of Social Security union official noted: 'I'm dealing with an increasing number of people suffering from stress-related illnesses. The trouble is, because you are only allowed 12 days sick leave, people are going to work when they are not really fit to do so' (cited *Guardian* 18 October 1995). As another official remarked:

> Our office sees the Social Fund as the 'sinbin', though there's nowhere nice to work in the Department of Social Security now . . . people who volunteered are fed up with the job . . . The reception-ists despise working on the Social Fund, they are terrified unless they can tell someone they've got a loan.
>
> (cited Craig 1988: 15)

The result is a high level of staff turnover and 'a high proportion of inexperienced trainees, temps [and] young recruits' (Howe 1985: 58) working on the front line of an increasingly embattled system.

## Demonising dependency

For many of those who rely financially upon the state the past twenty years have seen both a marked decline in their financial circumstances and a growing tension in their relationships with the system that is supposedly designed to support them. Financially, claimants have become poorer as, following the 1980 Social Security Acts, the annual uprating of benefits has failed to keep pace with the general increase in the standard of living. Like the working poor, they also have faced the disproportionately greater costs of increases in indirect taxation that have accompanied the reductions in income tax for the most wealthy. For some groups – such as the young, the unemployed – the fall in living standards has been even greater. Indeed it has been estimated that changes in government taxation and social-security policies were more important factors in the rapid growth of inequality during the 1980s than were the effects of recession or the changing nature of the labour market.

But the social-security system is more than just a system of income transfers. It is also a powerful institution in shaping wider perceptions of and ideas about poverty and in shaping the experience of those who depend upon it. During the past twenty years, although not for the first time, this dependency has been made into a problem: one that is opened up for public scrutiny and disapproval. The demonisation of the 'dependency culture' by which, as ever, dependence on state income is seen as demoralising and destructive of the incentives of the poor, although never of the rich, has focused attention not only on the costs that the system has to meet, but also on the moral character of those who are dependent.

In this process the motives and morality of the dependent poor have been opened up not only for public and media but also for official scrutiny (see *CARF* October/November 1998: 13). Suspicion has become the order of the day: the number and the range of activities of fraud investigators has been dramatically increased; telephone hotlines have been set up inviting the public to report on those thought to be cheating the system, at the same time as telephone hotlines introduced to help claimants claim benefit have been closed down.

Once again it is on the poorest that such activity has been concentrated. The introduction of the Social Fund following the 1986 Social Security Act exemplifies the pettiness in the application of regulations, the constant attention to minute detail and the lack of compassion within which this system operates. The cost-effectiveness of such strategies is dubious, but they are nevertheless pursued, regardless of the consequences for individual claimants. Officials are given targets to meet. The consequence has been to increase hostility between claimants and staff, and to add to the already stressful and demoralising experience of living in poverty the humiliation and degradation of being a claimant.

## Cheats and liars

The view of the Labour government's first Minister for Welfare Reform that the benefit system is 'steadily recruiting a nation of cheats and liars' (Field 1996: 11) is one that has always been attached to the social-security system. As Roy Sainsbury has argued, 'claimants who defraud the benefit system have always occupied a place among the demons of modern society' (Sainsbury 1998: 2), but in recent years this view has come to be both more publicly stated and backed by increasing legislation and other measures to detect supposed fraud and abuse. There is of course an important distinction between the two: whereas fraud is illegal, and carries with it the possibility of criminal sanction, concepts of abuse often extend to judgements about whether claimants 'really need' the benefits to which they are in fact legally entitled. It is, however, a distinction that is not always made, and as on the one hand drives to root out fraud have escalated, and, on the other, public questioning of the supposed 'dependency culture' has increased, so the two have mutually reinforced each other.

The claim that dishonesty within the benefit system is 'now on a massive scale' (Field 1996: 16) is one that needs to be treated carefully. Government estimates indicate that social-security fraud amounts to £1.6 billion: out of a total budget of nearly £100 billion, this, even if true, would be comparable to levels of fraudulent activity in most large firms and organisations. It is significantly less than the net loss to the public purse of the tax-free 'hidden economy', an economy estimated by the Inland Revenue at between £45 and £60 billion a year (Cook 1998: 11). Yet the estimates of social-security fraud are extremely unreliable.

In the first place, such estimates are based upon 'detected' fraud, the amount of which is then multiplied by 32 on the grounds that this is the number of weeks claims would have continued if the fraud had not been detected. But 'detected' fraud is also the product of a number of questionable factors. Thus claimants who, under investigation and the pressure of investigators, are frightened into withdrawing their claim will be added into the total, even though they may subsequently re-apply and have their claim legitimately reinstated. The Specialist Claims Control Units, established in the early 1980s but disbanded in 1986 following allegations that a number had intimidated and harassed claimants (*Poverty* 66 (1987)), have been only one in a series of initiatives in the drive against fraud. Amongst these, one of the most significant has been the setting of targets by the Benefits Agency, and the payment of its 5,500 fraud investigators on their performance in meeting or exceeding the targets. Curiously, these targets have always been met, including in 1996/7 when they were suddenly doubled from £680 million to £1,524 million. As an official working under similar performance-related pay for the Employment Service commented, 'every year we are given new targets – nationally, regionally and by sector – and every year the targets are miraculously obtained. That is because they are not real investigations' (cited *Guardian* 31 August 1995). According to one study, such incentives to detect fraud, and similar financial incentives given to local authorities for anti-fraud 'successes', have 'created an environment in which over-claiming the levels of benefit savings achieved has become endemic' (Sainsbury 1998: 6). Similarly the National Audit Office, in a scrutiny of fourteen local authorities in 1997, talked of 'possible sharp practice' and found reason to doubt the validity of 30 per cent of their alleged discoveries of fraud (ibid.). Yet it is on these practices that the estimates of fraud are based.

It is also these estimates that have been used to justify an increasingly strident campaign that has almost imperceptibly grouped together fraud, both on an organised criminal and small-scale individual level, 'scroungers', illegal immigrants, 'benefit tourists' and the undeserving poor. 'Those who think that this is a "something for nothing" society', argued Secretary of State for Social Security Peter Lilley in a Department of Social Security Press release (6 October 1993), 'can forget it. Benefits are rightly there for the needy, those who have paid towards them in taxes and contributions, not for people who think this country is a soft touch.' Frequently such campaigns have been justified in terms of protecting the interests of the 'honest claimants' as well as the general taxpayer, but according to a report in the *Sunday Times*, research commissioned by the Department of Social Security showed 'many Britons are surprisingly sympathetic towards bogus social security claimants [and] regarded social security cheats as poor and deserving rather than greedy' (*Sunday Times* 10 April 1994). In a survey conducted to test public opinion before launching a £750,000 advertising campaign to deter fraud and win public support for tougher measures, 28 per cent of respondents believed claimants defrauded the system because they needed more money; 14 per cent said the system did not provide enough to live on; only 6 per cent mentioned 'greed' (ibid.).

In 1995 the department launched a Five Year Security Strategy, at a cost of over £1 billion, to tackle the problem of fraud. The following year saw the closing down of the freephone benefits helpline, which had provided information to potential claimants on the benefits they could claim, and the opening of a freephone benefits 'cheatline', prominently advertised on billboard hoardings and in the newspaper press, which encouraged the public to inform on people suspected of cheating the system. In 1997 a Benefits Integrity Project was launched to investigate the claims of disabled people. This included the individual case, subsequently highlighted in the media in February 1998, of a widowed mother of two, deaf since birth and three-quarters paralysed following a spinal operation, whose benefit providing for overnight attendance was cut on the grounds that she had a catheter and therefore did not need assistance to go to the toilet at night. The fact that she had been claiming the allowance without, it was now argued, proper entitlement meant that the saving on her benefit would contribute towards the £1 billion total of fraudulent claims which ministers insisted the Benefits Integrity Project was aimed to recover. On the basis of this and other similar examples a *Guardian* editorial on 8 February 1998 spoke out: 'today it is not the Conservatives who are launching a class war against the poor . . . new Labour [has] connived in a disgraceful abuse of official statistics.' It is not of course simply the statistics that are abused in this process.

The 1997 Social Security Administration (Fraud) Act heralded another tightening of the mechanism by means of which claimants are supervised and those who fall foul of its rules are punished. The Act introduced a series of new offences, including dishonestly making a false statement, punishable on indictment by up to seven years' imprisonment or a fine or both, and failing to report a change in circumstances without reasonable excuse, which is now made a criminal offence. Changes of circumstance affect many people's lives, but for claimants the death of a dependent child, the beginning of a new relationship, or the frequent changes in the number of hours worked that are now common in the 'flexible' labour market are matters which, if unreported, are grounds for criminal prosecution. Prosecutions, even for government departments, are an expensive business, and where the amounts involved are relatively small, or where the evidence is considered to be weak, the Department of Social Security has generally preferred to 'persuade' claimants to terminate the claim or recover any overpaid benefit rather than go to court. Threats of prosecution, even where the evidence may not stand up in court, may be sufficient to lead claimants to withdraw their claims, especially when they are vulnerable, or where, as is usually the case, they lack knowledge of the rules and regulations covering the payment of benefit. As one such woman, accused of cohabiting with her boyfriend, recalled:

> The guy from the fraud squad just said that, as from today's date, [my boyfriend] now signs and claims for me and the two children . . . He suggested that if we did, then no further action would be taken, so that's what we did.
>
> (cited Rowlingson and Whyley 1998: 10)

The most-publicised examples of fraud involve those unemployed claimants who work unofficially in addition to claiming benefit. The scale of this practice is impossible to determine, although studies of the operation of the informal economy have frequently pointed out that the informal economy comprises a much greater proportion of those who are already in other paid jobs than it does unemployed benefit claimants. Those already in employment are much more likely to learn of opportunities for further informal work, and are more likely to have or to have access to the tools and equipment necessary to carry it out, than are the unemployed. Nevertheless, failure to declare earnings is subject to much greater scrutiny amongst claimants than it is amongst wage-earners. For governments concerned to reduce the cost to the exchequer of such illegal activities, the greater concentration on benefit fraud is, as a number of people have pointed out, anomalous: tax inspectors yield 108 times their salary in the money that they recover; the far greater number of social-security investigators save only 3 times their cost (*Independent* 26 October 1993).

Yet even if it is allowed that the number of people working while claiming benefit has increased substantially in recent years, the reasons for this are, as one social-security official pointed out, to be found in the growing inadequacy of the levels of benefit themselves: 'We're driving people into fraud because they can't possibly cope on the benefits so they have to disguise their circumstances' (cited Craig 1988: 15). In such circumstances, despite the fear that many claimants have of being caught, 'doing the double' is not seen as cheating the system; as one claimant pointed out, 'people aren't doing the double for fraud, they're doing it to exist' (cited Evason and Woods 1995: 49).

Research into those claimants who do work to supplement their benefits shows that the earnings of claimants 'were often extraordinarily low' (Evason and Woods 1995: 50). This included one claimant working for £17 a week for 15 hours' work; enough, she explained, to 'pay another bill'. Such exploitation, coupled with the complete absence of any employment rights or protection for those working illegally, is part of a market in which at least a number of employers are keen to operate. They know that 'claimants [have] no bargaining power and no option but to accept the wages offered' (ibid.). Nor is it clear that governments are willing or prepared to take effective measures to halt the situation. The risk of prosecution falls most heavily on claimants: while 182 claimants were prosecuted for working on the side in 1992/3, only seventeen employers were prosecuted for collusion (Evason and Woods 1995: 54). Yet if the motive for working on the side is survival, prosecution is unlikely to act as a deterrent: its consequence is simply to increase the vulnerability of those compelled to engage in it, while leaving largely intact an employment system that ekes out the inadequate benefits of the poor. As one claimant saw it, 'it's a vicious circle created by government. They can't control it – they don't even know if they want to control it' (cited Evason and Woods 1995: 51) .

## The new vitriol

There is a dreadful historical continuity to the abuse of the poorest and their presentation as something 'other' and inferior. This should be of no surprise given that such abuse is essential to the legitimation of persistent inequalities and the continued reproduction of poverty, especially in rich societies. The form the abuse has taken has changed over time, as have the legitimating explanations. But no matter what intellectual acrobatics have been deployed the central core of the explanation remains constant: society is not to blame. Poverty and destitution are primarily problems of individuals and families – they were failures and defective, whether through biology or socialisation, and in true Darwinian style they naturally drifted to the bottom of the social pile. Conversely, the rich were the cream, the most able and capable, and similarly floated to their natural position at the top.

Such arguments have historically been mobilised to explain not only poverty and the treatment of the poor but virtually every major form of social differentiation and injustice. They have been deployed forcefully to legitimate colonialism and the abuse of black people both in Britain and in its empire. They have been similarly used against women to justify their subordination in relation to men. They have been employed against people with physical disabilities, against those with learning difficulties, against gays and lesbians. Capitalist societies have an extraordinary history of taking differences between people and using and abusing them to maintain and sustain patterns of privilege and power.

Yet no matter how much attention and effort has been given to this reproduction of abusive human relationships, they have not gone without challenge. As Raymond Williams (1961) pointed out in *The Long Revolution*, human history is in large measure a history of people struggling to assert their humanity and rejecting subjugating categories that condemn them to being outside of the common weal. As a consequence, the history of domination is also a dialectical history of movement and counter-movement as excluded peoples have mobilised and struggled against ideologies and structures that condemn them to the margins. Real progress has been made as a consequence, not as a result of the compassion of the ruling elites or their enlightenment in view of new understandings, but in the face of unrelenting pressure from below and often of bitter resistance demanding heroic sacrifices (Kaye 1995: 96).

Nevertheless, as recent experience in Britain and the USA so clearly demonstrates, progress in these areas is by no means assured. This is particularly the case with respect to poverty and the poor. The past three decades have vividly demonstrated that there is no intrinsic compulsion in societies for the on-going amelioration of poverty and inequalities. Consequently, whilst it is possible to point to progress with respect to the formal civil and legal rights of women and black people, it is also evident that for many, their living standards and quality of life have significantly worsened. Blackness and poverty, for example, are now more closely correlated than ever before (Oppenheim 1993: 115). As Sivanandan observed:

> There has indeed been some sort of economic and social mobility for African-Caribbeans and Asians in the middle tranches of society. Equal opportunities and the Race Relations Act have worked for them. But, in the deprived and inner-city areas, on the dilapidated housing estates, in that third of society which has been socially and economically excluded for almost a generation, racism has got worse. There, racial attacks are on the increase, racial harassment is commonplace and fascism finds ready recruits. People who have defended their communities or themselves against such attacks, like Satpal Ram, are themselves arrested and arraigned – while the murders of promising youngsters like Stephen Lawrence and Manish Patel go unsolved and unpunished. And, in schools, young black boys are excluded at a rate four times higher than white boys.
>
> (Sivanandan 1998: 73)

Raup, an American criminologist, has noted how this deterioration is not only the result of unemployment and the growth in low-paid and casualised employment, but also a consequence of the new politics of hatred and abuse associated with more vitriolic depictions of the poor: 'Though black Americans have long struggled beneath the weight of dominant ideologies, the term "black underclass" has done much more than past ideologies to dehumanise inner-city blacks' (Raup 1996: 163). This dehumanisation is the handmaiden of neglect and new forms of brutalisation. It has eclipsed the rhetoric of the social-democratic welfare state with its notions of entitlement, rehabilitation and treatment and replaced it with a politics and practice of repression, hatred and studied neglect. In Britain, we have witnessed the creation of a political culture where the poor can be freely disparaged. Barbara Amiel typified this perspective when she argued in the *Sunday Times* that the time had now come to rid society of its compassionate impulses which she held responsible for the creation of 'the underclass'. She also exemplifies a new confidence amongst the elites in expressing in public and in writing what many may have thought in the past but felt restrained from making known:

> In summary: we cannot deport people who are now here. But we can segregate the underclass and forget about egalitarian principles. We should try to reintroduce the best of our values while getting rid of the worst. We must stop ruining our free society by enacting rules appropriate for a zoo. Just because some of the rooms in our house have been taken over by pigs and donkeys does not mean we should turn the entire kingdom into a place appropriate for the housing of animals.
>
> (cited Rose 1996: 338–9)

This new and often racist vitriol towards the poorest in society marks an alarming shift. It is the vocabulary of legitimation for a new set of arrangements to manage the widening disparities in wealth, income and life chances which the elites are seizing upon while progressive and working-class organisations are in disarray. These arrangements embody the view that there are whole clusters of the population who are superfluous and no longer required in either the short or the long term. As Nick Davies observed:

> They are in the deepest sense redundant. Looking at them from a strictly economic point of view, these former workers and their families are worthless. More than that, they are an expensive burden – at least they will be if they are to be properly housed and clothed and fed, if they are to be given decent schools and hospitals. So, why bother? . . . From an economic point of view, they are worth nothing, they will be given the bare minimum. For these redundant humans, the creation of poverty is the final solution.
>
> (Davies 1997: 299–300)

As a consequence, we now witness the re-emergence of studied neglect whereby the very poorest are increasingly corralled in housing estates and neighbourhoods which take on ever more characteristics of the most impoverished regions of the world. Accompanying this has been a rapid increase in the use of prisons and the penal system to replace social welfare as a means of controlling the poor and the consequences of their poverty. In both Britain and the USA the 1990s have seen dramatic increases in the prison population. Since coming to power in 1992, Clinton has overseen a 50 per cent growth in the prison population from 1.2 to 1.8 million. In total 6 million Americans are under the supervision of the criminal justice system – in prison, on probation, awaiting trial or on the run, including 40 per cent of all young blacks in Washington DC (*Observer* 8 February 1998). A similar trajectory is evident in Britain, with the prison population at new record levels of nearly 64,000 having risen from 40,000 in just over five years (ibid.). With the British prison population increasing by 1,000 a month at the time of writing, it is now estimated that a new prison is required every fortnight. According to the *Observer* columnist Nick Cohen, 'it is not too fanciful to talk of a prison state in the land of the free'. He continued: 'New Labour says it wants to imitate Clinton's success in reducing unemployment. It doesn't seem to understand that Clinton is keeping the jobless figures low by jailing the poor instead of supporting them' (*Observer* 8 February 1998).

To read the mass-circulation newspapers one would imagine that prisons are full of the most heinous and dangerous criminals. But as the *New Internationalist* points out, this is not the case:

> The vast majority of matters dealt with by the criminal justice system are non violent, often petty. Prostitution, drug offences, non payment of fines, car theft, social security fraud, loitering, curfew violations, shop-lifting: all these often end in prison sentences (sometimes quite long ones). *Criminal justice is being used to keep an increasingly desperate underclass from cheating to survive.*
>
> (*New Internationalist* August 1996: 24–5; emphasis added)

Over the past twenty years successive Home Secretaries in Britain have denied any causal link between increasing poverty and crime, despite mounting evidence to the contrary. At the same time the riots and disturbances that have punctuated urban life have been explained away as having nothing whatsoever to do with social conditions and everything to do with problematic individuals and communities. After the Handsworth riots in Birmingham in September 1985, then Home Secretary Douglas Hurd declared that they were 'not social phenomena but crimes' (cited Rose 1996: 96), while in his characteristically brazen fashion Michael Howard argued that 'we should have no truck with trendy theories that try to explain away crime by blaming socio-economic factors' (cited Rose 1996: 92). In contrast a report in 1994 by the Catholic Bishops' Social Welfare Committee, entitled *A Time For Justice*, echoing earlier concerns expressed by the Archbishop of Canterbury about 'deep social divisions', went on to argue:

> There is strong evidence of a relationship between unemployment

and crime, especially at a time of growing inequalities of income . . . Present-day western society places a high premium on material success, but we have seen an increasingly unequal distribution of the legitimate means to reach that goal. Some unfortunately adopt illegitimate methods instead . . . Reductions in social security payments for many claimants, and the withdrawal of benefit from 16- to 17-year old people, place many under severe financial pressure, and increase the temptation to resort to petty crime as a way out of destitution or overwhelming financial problems.

(cited *Independent* 14 April 1994)

Noting 'the ineffectiveness of prison in rehabilitation, its damaging and counter-productive effects and high costs' it also went on to argue that 'the length of prison sentences imposed on many offenders is excessive in comparison with those of other countries and it has been steadily increasing over recent years' (ibid.). It also felt fit to remark on the bias within the criminal justice system which meant that the poorest were likely to be dealt with hardest:

It is quite clear that there is a relationship between people's status and the likelihood of their suffering the more extreme penalties prescribed by the law. To be homeless and vagrant may attract a criminal penalty which would not be visited on, say, financial failure or bankruptcy higher up the social scale.

(cited *Guardian* 14 April 1994)

While the poor have been increasingly criminalised, at the same time their ability to defend themselves has been steadily whittled away. In the wake of a barrage of Conservative measures, including the removal of the right to silence, New Labour within its first year of office has made significant changes to the legal-aid system. On the spurious grounds of equity, the Lord Chancellor claimed that changes were needed because they privileged the poor in their access to justice and 'this should not go on' (*CARF* December/January 1998: 7). Yet in reforming legal aid, the Labour government has not only abandoned the key welfare principle that legal aid, like the health service, was to be 'free at the point of need and equally accessible to all' (ibid.). It has also removed a significant resource to those who want to challenge injustices in that legal aid was available to challenge landlords, the abuse of police powers and medical negligence amongst other things. As with the penal system in general the reform of legal aid will fall hardest on those with the least. According to *CARF*,

The Labour government like the Clinton administration in the US wants to appear modern and to speak the language of rights, so long as the rights are cultural and not class based . . . The rights of asylum seekers, immigrants, those charged with criminal offences . . . carry less weight to a government obsessed with law and order, whose priority is to retain the votes of the business community and of 'middle England'.

(*CARF* January 1998: 9)

For the dispossessed imprisonment epitomises their abandonment as human beings. The conditions in which they are housed, their vulnerability to arbitrary violence and abuse, are symptomatic of their perceived worthlessness. In addition, the growth of prisons is having a devastating impact on young black men, many caught in a pincer of poverty leading to crime in order to survive and deep-rooted racism which condemns them to being seen as irredeemable. What Marable notes for the US is equally true for Britain:

The racial oppression that defines US society as a whole is most dramatically apparent within the criminal justice system and the prisons. Today, about one-half of all inmates in prisons and jails – or more than three quarters of a million people – are African-American.

(Marable 1997: 44)

In Britain black people are seven times more likely to be imprisoned than white people: 547 per 100,000 compared with 77 per 100,000 for whites in England and Wales (*Guardian* 9 April 1994).

For black people of course racism compounds the abuse of the poor, amongst whom they are represented in disproportionate numbers. In addition black people are subjected to the increasing internal controls that have come with the dismantling of the welfare state. Take the 1996 Asylum and Immigration Act and its accompanying social-security regulations which removed benefits from asylum seekers once their claim had been rejected by the Home Office. This punitive legislation was introduced following a government-fuelled media panic that the country was being overwhelmed by bogus asylum seekers attracted to Britain by its supposedly generous benefit allowances. Whilst seemingly focused on a specific section of the population, the Act is of much broader significance, both in terms of reinforcing the message that the state is not driven by humanitarian concerns and in its negative implications for race relations. The Act itself removed rights to child benefit and to local-authority housing for immigrants 'of a class to be specified by the minister'. It also introduced criminal sanctions for employers found to be employing people who have entered or remained in the country illegally. As *Statewatch* noted, the impact of the Act on asylum seekers is severe and will inevitably bear down on all people who appear 'foreign', especially black people:

> The [Act's] employer sanctions will effectively deter most small employers – except the most unscrupulous ones – from employing black or foreign labour. They will not want the bother of checking passports and national insurance numbers; safer just to say 'no blacks'. There will be no work. And there will be no public housing, no child benefit – not even for the children of 'immigrants' who have been living, working and paying taxes and national insurance in Britain for over 20 years. The measures are bound to result, not only in more poor black people living on the streets, a sight which will be seized upon by race-card politicians of all political colours by whipping up yet more popular racism, but also in more suicides as the means of life are taken from those with nothing.
>
> (*Statewatch* November/December 1995: 18)

In the USA we are seeing new brutalisms as an increasing number of states introduce 'three strikes and out' measures which condemn offenders to a lifetime in prison with no hope of parole, and the growing use of the death penalty, which has every possibility of being extended as the costs of imprisonment increase (Shichor and Sechrest (eds) 1996). In the process, the notion that prisons are only for the worthless is reinforced and the public is further exposed to the idea that the only response to such a threat from within is through the most pitiless of punishments.

This increasing use of prisons in both Britain and America, like the onslaught on welfare entitlements, is part and parcel of the new politics of pessimism and repression by which we are encouraged to understand the most impoverished and vulnerable as being beyond redemption and their position in society as an accurate reflection of their worthlessness. We are encouraged in this thinking by endless rounds of scapegoating and demonisation in which specific groups are highlighted for castigation and rejection. In all of these discourses that of racism is never far from the surface, and in attacks on lone-parent families in the USA, and on young male offenders in both Britain and America, has been explicit. The consequences are however consistent in suggesting particularities instead of similarities, of focusing attention downwards rather than upwards. As Sklar has argued:

Racist and sexist scapegoating make it easier to forget that the majority of poor people are white. Scapegoating makes it easier to treat inner-city neighbourhoods like outsider cities – separate, unequal and disposable. Scapegoating encourages people to think of 'the poor' as the 'Other America'. Them and not Us. That makes it easier to divide people who should be working together to transform harmful social and economic policies; makes it easier to write off more and more Americans as Untouchables; makes it easier to leave unjust economic practices untouched.

Many white men who are 'falling down' the economic ladder are being encouraged to believe they are falling because women and people of colour are climbing over them to the top or dragging them down from the bottom. That way they will blame women and people of colour rather than the system.

(Sklar 1995: 117)

These are miserable times when those at the very bottom of society are being abused on so many fronts. It as if a decision has been made to abandon up to one-third of the population as surplus to requirements both now and in the foreseeable future. The preferred course of action is the reduction of state services and resources to the barest minimum which in turn are then made more difficult (and humiliating) to access. However, if the poor should cause trouble to the mainstream when they leave their now more ghettoised neighbourhoods and estates, then the state is more prepared and tooled up to intervene, with prisons and the criminal justice system at the forefront. When this happens, as has been illustrated in the case of so many black men who have died in police custody, the state acts with little regard for their civil liberties. For as David Rose observed at the very end of his book on law and order:

Underclass, *untermensch*. What price due process when an entire class is guilty? Why should it matter if their convictions are safe and satisfactory? Where better to segregate them than in prison?

It is a glimpse into hell: the 30/30/40 society mediated by violence, with all pretence of equality before the law removed. It must not come to pass.

(Rose 1996: 339)

# 4 The vile maxim of the masters

[Adam] Smith's admiration for individual enterprise was tempered still
further by his contempt for 'the vile maxim of the masters of mankind':
'All for ourselves, and nothing for other people.'

(Chomsky 1993: 19)

In his *Essays in Persuasion*, John Maynard Keynes described capitalism
as that 'extraordinary belief that the nastiest of men for the nastiest of
motives will somehow work for the benefit of all'.

(Hewlett 1993: 51)

For the poor, life under capitalism has always been short and, for the
most part, brutish. The poorer people are, the less long they will live, the
more disease they will suffer and the more stunted will be their lives
than those of the rich. Currently this is reflected in the fact that in
Britain infant mortality is almost four times higher amongst the poorest than it is amongst the richest of the population, while once beyond
childhood, life expectancy is cut short by some seven or eight years.
Although these consequences have only been reliably measured for the
past 100 years, it has always been thus. That this is well known – and
there are volumes of research, both official and unofficial, that document the consequences of poverty – does not make any difference.
Although capitalism has shown itself capable of reform, of alleviating
the consequences, but not removing the causes, of poverty, social
reform has never been prompted by the simple fact of poverty. Rather
it has been the calculation of the threat that poverty poses to wealth,
and of what is necessary to remove this threat while maintaining existing relationships, that has informed the development of state policy.
    British (or, more accurately, English) capitalism has a particularly
ruthless history, both globally – in its history of colonisation, including

its near neighbours in Wales, Ireland and Scotland – and within the confines of its own nation state. The 'making' of its working class was a long drawn-out, and continuing, process stretching over many centuries. The expropriation and dispossession of the peasantry and its transformation into a potential class of wage-earners formed a central part of this process. But a working class is made not only through the disruption and destruction of older forms of economic and social relationships: the denial of alternative means of subsistence other than wage labour. A working class is also constituted, and daily reconstituted, as a working class only through the creation of a whole set of relationships and ideologies which proclaim this condition – and the poverty which results – as natural or at least inevitable. In both these processes, violence has been a constant feature.

The break-up of feudalism that marked the origins of capitalism in Britain was, in economic terms, itself a bloody affair. The enclosure of land, the eviction at least of the smaller peasantry and tenant farmers, and the break-up and dismissal of the large feudal households and armies created a class of dispossessed and propertyless people: 'a new class of men, henceforward described by the legislature under the denomination of Poor' (Eden 1796: 57). The pace of this transformation was varied: beginning in parts of England in the Middle Ages, it was not, for example, to be completed in Scotland until the ruthless destruction of the Highland Clearances in the eighteenth century, when thousands were forcibly moved off the land on which they had gained their living (Prebble 1969).

However, at least in its early pre-industrial development, capitalism could not be assured that those who had lost the means to support themselves would necessarily and meekly follow a path to the labour market. Even as late as the end of the nineteenth century Sidney and Beatrice Webb, the founding members of the Fabian Society, would complain that 'the able bodied men . . . were supposed to be face to face with the alternatives of either working or starving. As a matter of fact our social organisation is still too loose to narrow their choice to any such extent' (Webb and Webb 1929: 394). Before then, however, and in a pre-industrial and predominantly rural society, alternatives to wage labour in the form of begging, charity, banditry or simply settling on unoccupied and common land were many. To drive the poor into the developing market for labour was to call on the power of the state and the development of a series of Poor Laws that have left an indelible mark on the economic, social and psychological face of the nation.

Thus in 1349 the Statute of Labourers, the first of the English Poor Laws, ordered

> That every man and woman of our realm of England . . . not living
> in merchandise, nor exercising any craft, nor having of his own
> whereof he may live, nor proper land . . . and not serving any other,
> shall be bounden to serve him which so shall him require.
>
> (23 Edward III, cited de Schweinitz 1947: 28)

Over the following 200 years the penalty imposed on the poor for loitering, vagabondage and begging – in short, for refusing to work –
increased to hysterical proportions. In 1531 an 'Act Concerning the
Punishment of Beggars and Vagabonds' ordered that anyone 'being
strong and able in their bodies to work' should be 'tied to the end of a
cart naked and be beaten with whips till his body be bloody' (22 Henry
VIII c12, cited ibid.). Five years later, the penalty for a second offence
of 'loitering, wandering and idleness' was increased so that the
offender should be 'not only whipped again, but also shall have the
upper part of the gristle of his right ear clean cut off' (27 Henry VIII
c25, cited ibid.), while in the reign of Edward VI in 1547 it was ordered
that 'If any man or woman, able to work, should refuse to labour, and
live idly for three days, that he or she should be branded with a red-hot
iron on the breast with the letter V, and should be adjudged the slave,
for two years, of any person who should inform against such an idler'
(cited ibid.). Any attempt to escape during this period would make
that person a slave for life, while a second attempted escape would
mean that he or she 'shall have judgement to suffer pains and execution
of death as a felon and as enemies of the Commonwealth' (1 Edward
VI c3, cited ibid.).

In these ways the social violence of the state was harnessed to the
economic violence that had created the problem of poverty. As Marx
noted, the creation of a propertyless class had made it

> dependent on the sale of its labour capacity or on begging,
> vagabondage and robbery as its only source of income . . . It is a
> matter of historic record that they tried the latter first, but were
> driven from this path by gallows, stocks and whippings onto the
> narrow road to the labour market; owing to this fact, the govern-
> ments of Henry VII, VIII, etc. appear as conditions of the historic
> dissolution process and as makers of the conditions for the exis-
> tence of capital.
>
> (Marx 1973: 507)

The early Poor Laws were only one instrument through which the
power of the state was used to create the conditions for the growth of

capitalism. Capital requires labour, and while the enclosure of common land, which reached dizzying heights through successive Acts of Parliament during the eighteenth century, was to produce a growing propertyless population, the existence of alternatives to wage labour – the 'looseness of social organisation' that the Webbs referred to – would also need to be curtailed. The Parliamentary Select Committee on Criminal Commitments and Convictions in 1827 highlighted just one such example:

> In the immediate vicinity of the dwellings of such half-starved labourers there are abundantly-stocked preserves of game, in which, during a single night, these dissatisfied young men can obtain a rich booty by snaring hares or taking and killing pheasants . . . offences which they cannot be brought to acknowledge to be any violation of private property.
>
> (cited Hammond and Hammond 1913: 191)

The infamous Game Laws, by which the right to hunt game was restricted to those with property, imposed a penalty of seven years' penal transportation on anyone found in illegal possession of nets. Between 1805 and 1833 criminal convictions increased more than five-fold, with one in seven convictions taking place under the Game Laws. Thus the aristocratic and ruling elite were assured of their favourite pastimes of hunting, shooting and fishing, while the poor found yet another alternative source of subsistence closed down.

In a myriad of ways the naked power of the state was used to further the interests of those alone who controlled and managed it. But violence in this form and of this order could not be sustained indefinitely. Above all it could not erase the sense of injustice that it, and the system that created it, produced. As Joseph Arch, one of the leaders of the agricultural workers' 'revolt' of 1872 recounted:

> Those who owned and held the land believed, and acted up to their belief as far as they were able, that the land belonged to the rich man only, that the poor had no part or lot in it, and had no sort of claim on society. If the poor man dared to marry and have children, they thought he had no right to claim the necessary food wherewith to keep himself and his family alive. They thought, too, every mother's son of them, that when a labourer could no longer work he had lost the right to live. Work was all they wanted from him; he was to work and hold his tongue, year in and year out, early and late, and if he could not work, why, what was the use of him? It was

what he was made for, to labour and toil for his betters, without complaint on a starvation wage.

(cited Hollis 1973: 122)

Although the coercive power of the state remained, to this day, to underpin the incentive to work, it was the seemingly impersonal hand of the market that, as it developed, was left to bring the poor into line. As J. Townsend argued in 'A Dissertation on the Poor Laws' in 1786:

There must be a degree of pressure, and that which is attended with the least violence will be the best. When hunger is either felt or feared, the desire of obtaining bread will quietly dispose the mind to undergo the greatest hardships, and will sweeten the severest labours . . . The wisest legislature will never be able to devise a more equitable, a more effectual, or in any respect a more suitable punishment than hunger is for a disobedient servant.

(cited Poynter 1969: xvi)

Hunger, at least in the modern world, is not of course a natural phenomenon, but the result of a particular form of economic and social organisation. So too is the market. Its presentation as an inevitable feature of human society obscures its social origins. Yet it is a powerful weapon. By the end of the eighteenth century, on the eve of the industrial revolution, market forces were to complete the process that would drive the poor into the factories and mills. Falling agricultural wages and rising prices left no alternative. As one contemporary observed:

Formerly many of the lower sort of people occupied tenements of their own, with parcels of land about them. On these they raised a considerable part of their subsistence, without being obliged, as now, to buy all they want at shops. But [now] they are crowded together in decayed farmhouses with hardly enough ground about them for a cabbage garden, and being thus reduced to mere hirelings, they are very liable to come to want.

(cited Hasbach 1908: 129)

To be reduced to mere hirelings is the essence of labour under capitalism. Its achievement in Britain, on a scale unparalleled at the time in any other country, was one of the decisive factors that enabled the British ruling class to pioneer the transition to industrial capitalism. Another was the availability of a mass of surplus capital for investment in new machinery and factories. This book cannot do full justice to the story of where this wealth came from, or the human consequences that the gaining of it had: the conquest and pillage of India, the extermination of millions of indigenous people across the globe and the pauperisation of many millions more, the inhumanity of the slave trade in which Britain excelled – all reveal the vile maxim of those for whom wealth and power over-rode any recognition of a common humanity. It is a story of brutality and indifference which, even before the added power of industrial might was to make the British empire the largest in the world, was to establish capitalism as a global force and to feed its insatiable appetite for the fruits of human toil.

Industrialisation was to turn the beast into a monster. Factories swallowed up the lives and limbs of men, women and children, and spat them out, merely to be replaced by more. Market forces (that combination of economic and social relationships, of hunger and legislation, that left no alternative) ensured a constant supply of 'hands'. But the physical creation of a working class could not alone ensure its compliance with, still less its acceptance of, a system so disrespectful of human life.

## Constructing social policy

During the course of the nineteenth century the attempt was to be made to construct a social policy that would proclaim the social relationships of industrial capitalism as natural and inevitable, and secure the conditions for its long-term viability. This construction would not only have to contend with alternative understandings of human relationships and visions of a different social order within the working class. It would also have to confront elements within the British ruling class itself. A ruling class, like capitalism itself, is never the pure expression of one particular interest. Just as capitalism has transformed and built upon but never wholly eradicated pre-capitalist forms of economic and social organisation – the institution of the family, or slavery, for example – so its ruling class embodies both the dominant representatives of industrial and financial capital and those representatives of older forms of power. In Britain, whose ruling class has remained in power for centuries – unchallenged, if not untroubled, by the revolutions and coups that have marked the development of other capitalist societies – this fusion of old, landed aristocratic wealth, of mercantile and financial capital, with newer forms of industrial capital has given a particular imprint to its cultural and class relationships.

Britain, despite New Labour's attempts in the 1990s to rebrand it as a 'young country', is in fact a very old country, its sedimented layers of power and privilege, of ideologies, beliefs and attitudes contributing to its distinctiveness as a social formation. While the historical continuity of the British ruling class, and its ability to accommodate newcomers without risking its own demise, has been one of its greatest strengths this does not mean that it has been without difficulty. The construction of social policy in the nineteenth century was thus to reflect some of these tensions: the differing conceptions of social order represented by an old feudal aristocracy on the one hand and a new industrial bour-geoisie on the other; their differing attitudes towards poverty and the poor. Added to these have been tensions, and conflicts of interest, between big and small capital, finance versus industry, the short-term goals of a quick profit as against the long-term goals of economic and political stability. These tensions are the meat of political struggle: of struggle not only between the rulers and the ruled, but within the ruling class itself, and the state is the site where the struggle has most often been played out, reflecting the interests of the most powerful and dom-inant factions while at the same time attempting to secure the collective rule of the whole.

The construction of social policy that took place during the nine-teenth century – the vastly increased power and role of the state that took place despite repeated claims to a principle of laissez-faire – cen-tred upon the reformulation of the Poor Law. Two years after the Great Reform Act of 1832, whereby the old aristocratic elite finally recognised the power of the industrial bourgeoisie and granted it a share in polit-ical power, the Poor Law Amendment Act was brought into being. More popularly known, at least amongst those at whom it was directed, as the Poor Man's Destruction Act or the Starvation Law, this one piece of legislation was to dominate state policy towards the poor – was effectively to be the state's social policy – for the rest of the century. It was in relation to and often in tandem with it that subsequent develop-ments of policy would take place during the first half of the twentieth century, and, although finally repealed in 1948, its principles remained at the core of the welfare state.

Drawing on the newly established 'science' of political economy, with its seemingly immutable 'laws' of supply and demand, the 1834 Poor Law directly repudiated the claim that those made dependent on wage labour had a right either to work or to be provided with relief when work was not available. Instead it offered conditional relief to the des-titute subject to the principle of less eligibility: 'that his situation on the whole shall not be made really or apparently so eligible as the situation of the independent labourer of the lowest class' (Checkland and Checkland (eds) 1974: 335). The mechanism to achieve this was to be the workhouse test. As the Poor Law Commission which drew up the report recognised, making the condition of those relieved less eligible than the condition of the lowest-paid independent labourer was difficult, if not impossible, when many of those in work failed to earn enough to live on. The problem would be overcome by requiring those seeking assistance to give up their freedom, to be separated from their wives, husbands and children, to put on the pauper's uniform and to enter the strictly disciplined workhouse, where they would, after a manner, be clothed, fed and sheltered, but where they would lose all civil rights. The workhouse would thus act as a 'test' of destitution, deterring those who were not wholly destitute from applying for help, and exerting a constant pressure on its inmates to re-enter the labour market at whatever cost. As the report noted approvingly, the effects of the workhouse were transformatory:

> New life, new energy is infused into the constitution of the pauper; he is like one aroused from sleep, his relations with all his neighbours, high and low, is changed; he surveys his former employers with new eyes. He begs a job . . .
>
> (Checkland and Checkland (eds) 1974: 358)

Driving those who could work back into the labour market was only one consequence of the 'new' Poor Law. For the most part, and except at times of economic depression and high unemployment, when it was in any case incapable of dealing with the large numbers involved, the workhouse test was to be applied to the working-class elderly, the sick, widowed, single mothers and the disabled; its harshness justified as a necessary incentive, even for these groups, to make their own provision through thrift and savings against such an eventuality. That most were unable to do so did not defeat the Poor Law's objectives. The stigma of the Poor Law was not intended to exercise its transformatory effects only on those who claimed relief, but also, and crucially, on the attitudes and behaviour of the poor as a whole. As Sir George Nicholls, whose pioneering use of a deterrent workhouse in the parish of Southwell in Nottinghamshire provided the model for reform and earned him the appointment as Commissioner to implement the new national regime, argued, 'I wish to see the Poor House looked to with dread by the labouring classes, and the reproach for being an inmate of it extend down from father to son . . . For without this, where is the needful stimulus to industry?' (cited Poynter 1969: 314).

The stigmatisation of state assistance, and its modelling on principles of deterrence and punishment, would thus act as a necessary adjunct to the labour market, a fact well-recognised by the working-class move-ment of the time. As one workers' newspaper recognised:

> Once adopt the principle that whatever may be the labourer's con-dition, the pauper's must still be a degree worse, and that moment you place the labourer at the utter mercy of the capitalist – you compel him, in fact, to take whatever wages he is offered; for if he refuses, he has no other recourse than to go where he is to be less comfortable still. Twist and turn the proposition as you may, it inevitably comes to this – its adoption places the 'independent' labourer at the utter mercy of his employer.
>
> (*Poor Man's Guardian* 14 November 1835)

Or as the *Northern Star* put it, 'thus "Philosophy" accomplished its aims. It got at the wages of labour' (cited Hollis 1973: 212).

## Remoralising the poor

That the reform of the Poor Law did not lead to the simple abolition of all relief from the state, as a number of contemporaries had argued it should, is significant. Considerations of political stability aside, the more astute reformers recognised the value, indeed the necessity, of a state policy that could shape attitudes and relationships. 'We saw', said George Nicholls, 'that it compelled them, *bred* them, to be industrious, sober, provident, careful of themselves, of their parents and children' (cited Poynter 1969: 315). The market alone was insufficient to achieve this, and despite popularised claims of 'laissez-faire' – of the principle that the state should not intervene – the reality was that the creation of the necessary attitudes towards work and poverty required the active intervention of the state. Amongst the more sophisticated political economists, those who directed the growth of state policy during the nineteenth century, this was self-evident. 'The social body', argued James Kay-Shuttleworth, who would be the driving force behind the development of state schooling for the working class,

> cannot be constructed like a machine, on abstract principles which merely include physical motions, and their numerical results in the production of wealth . . . Political economy, though its object be to ascertain the means of increasing the wealth of nations, cannot accomplish its designs, without at the same time regarding the cul-tivation of religion and morality.
>
> (Kay-Shuttleworth 1832: 64)

The moralisation of the working class – the creation of a particular set of beliefs, attitudes and behaviour concerning the inevitability of poverty, the need for independence and the naturalness of the market – was the over-riding purpose of state policy. The mechanisms required to do this, the creation of a national, uniform system and a powerful centralised agency of the state to enforce it, met with considerable opposition, not least from the working-class movement which, and especially in the industrialised North of England, successfully resisted the implementation of the new Poor Law until well into the second half of the nineteenth century. But opposition was also found within the ruling class itself: from those who opposed any form of state activity as an infringement on the absolute sanctity of private property, as well as the smaller number of those whose lingering attachment to the paternalistic order of feudal control, where the rich owed an obligation to the poor so long as the poor stayed in their place, led them to recoil at what they saw as the barbarism and potentially divisive effects of the new system. The latter, personified in the Justices of the Peace who had for some 300 years overseen the operation of the old Poor Law, 'not wisely, indeed, or beneficially, but still with benevolent and honest intentions . . . the mischief they have done was, in part, the necessary consequence of their social position' (Checkland and Checkland (eds) 1974: 290), were effectively removed from office, 'left', according to Nassau Senior, one of the principal authors of the report, 'either excluded from influence in the management of their own parishes, or forced to accept a seat in the Board of Guardians, and to debate and vote among shopkeepers and farmers' (cited Levy 1970: 87). As for the former, 'who are so blind to the true interests of their own order', argued Kay-Shuttleworth, 'I am not willing to screen them from just contempt'; their protestations were to be over-ruled in an alliance between state policy makers and

> the enlightened manufacturers of the country, acutely sensible to the miseries of large masses of the operative body . . . ranked amongst the foremost advocates of every measure . . . and the most active promoters of every plan which can conduce to their physical improvement or their moral elevation.
>
> (Kay-Shuttleworth 1832: 10)

## Social reform

By the end of the nineteenth century the British ruling class was once again to face the necessity of social reform. 'It looks', argued one contemporary,

> as if we were in the presence of one of those periodic upheavals in the labour world such as occurred in 1833-4, and from time to time since that date, each succeeding occurrence showing a marked advance in organisation on the part of the workers and the necessity for a corresponding change of tactics on the part of the employers.
>
> (cited Winter 1974: 27)

Conditions at the end of the nineteenth century were of course substantially different than they had been at the beginning: the growth of working-class organisation advancing with urbanisation and industrialisation, with the spread of specifically socialist and, although in a minority, revolutionary ideologies, and the rise of a new, militant trades unionism. That this was to take place in the midst of a collapse in global capitalism that marked the first 'great depression', and a crisis of British imperialism sparked by the colonial advances of newly industrialised countries such as Germany was what called for a corresponding change of tactics. By the outbreak of the first world war, state policy was to be substantially reformulated, although key continuities were to remain.

Social reform, nevertheless, was to be slow in coming. From the outbreak of the great depression, with its rising levels of unemployment and poverty, in the early 1870s, it was to be over thirty years before decisive action was taken. As Kay-Shuttleworth had noted earlier, 'general efforts are seldom made for the relief of partial ills until they threaten to convulse the whole social condition' (Kay-Shuttleworth 1832: 18). It was only when this threat became unavoidable that a far-reaching programme of reform was introduced: by 1905 little had been done, six years later the state had introduced a system of National Insurance for health and unemployment benefits, old-age pensions, school meals and medical inspections, a regulation of the labour market and minimum wages in certain industries. It was a radical, though by no means revolutionary, programme of reform, designed to strengthen capitalism in the face of the challenges it faced. 'That', after all, argued one advocate, 'is the doctrine of reformers. We seek to cleanse, to repair, to strengthen private property' (Arnold 1888: 569).

Central to this task was the attempt to draw a sharp distinction within the working class between the 'genuinely unemployed' and 'respectable' workers on the one hand, deserving of more positive state assistance, and the undeserving 'residuum' – the exact equivalent of today's so-called 'underclass' – whose poverty was seen as the result of their own fecklessness, and for whom a punitive Poor Law was to continue as the only appropriate response. The drawing of this distinction reflected the new political preoccupations of Britain's ruling class. Previously, and as far back as the sixteenth century, demarcations had been made between what might have been called the deserving and undeserving poor, but then the distinction had been between those who could not work and those who could, the impotent and the able-bodied. Now the lines were to be redrawn, based not on physical status and ability but on supposed moral character. In place of the deserving elderly or sick and the undeserving unemployed came the deserving unemployed and elderly, and their undeserving counterparts.

That the redrawing of this distinction coincided with the challenge of organised labour was of course no accident. In the flood of social surveys and investigation prompted by the rise of social unrest from the 1870s onwards, what was revealed, to many for the first time, was that the working class was not a homogeneous group, an undifferentiated mass of labour-power, but was stratified according to levels of skill, organisation and consciousness. Typically, at the bottom, were placed 'the great industrial residuum of all the industrial classes of the community, the men who have failed in life, or who, through feebleness of physique, or through want of perseverance or some hereditary incapacity, have not even succeeded in failing' (Fabian Society 1886: 4). In an article entitled 'The industrial residuum', Helen Bosanquet considered the implications of their position:

> Taking this type of character as one of our data, we may now ask about its effects upon the economic position of its possessor. It will be found to result invariably in his permanent failure to maintain himself (and those legally dependent upon him) in that standard of comfort which is considered necessary, and insisted upon by the community.
>
> (Bosanquet 1893: 604)

With such a prognosis, there was little to be done, short of penal incarceration, sterilisation or other often-suggested measures to bring their lives to an end. As William Beveridge, the later 'founder' of the post-war welfare state, saw it:

> The line between independence and dependence, between the effi-
> cient and the unemployable, has to be made clearer and broader . . .
> [the latter] must become the acknowledged dependants of the State,
> removed from industry and maintained adequately in public insti-
> tutions; but with complete and permanent loss of all citizen rights –
> including not only the franchise, but civil freedom and fatherhood.
>
> (Beveridge 1906: 327)

At the other end of the spectrum were what Charles Booth described
as 'the higher class of labour and the best paid of the artisans . . . the
non-commissioned officers of the industrial army' (Booth 1904: 53), or
as other writers saw them:

> Protected against the chances and changes of his environment by
> his 'social habit', he has accumulations of property and cash, he
> has relatives and friends beholden to him: he is specially preferred
> by a particular foreman or master as a reliable desirable servant.
>
> (Jackson and Pringle 1909: 119)

'It is here', added Booth ominously, 'we find the springs of socialism
and revolution' (1904: 308). Or as another social investigator reported:
'the most advanced section seeks to get rid of the state itself and aims
at self-governing social organisation' (Anon 1889: 264).

The redrawing of the distinction between the deserving and the undeserving was crucially to attempt to keep the two apart. Evidence of the
consequences of the failure to do this had already become apparent in
the Trafalgar Square riots of 1886 when unemployed demonstrators
had invaded the west end of London attacking the fashionable clubs of
the rich and looting their shops. As one contemporary observer
recalled, 'at first the majority were shiftless flotsam and jetsam of the
community, [but] day by day the numbers increased of the more
respectable workmen . . . The mob had now become articulate and
capable of suggesting methods of extending the existing system of
relief' (Burleigh 1887: 773).

From the point of view of the maintenance of social order, the very
poor have always been seen more as a nuisance than a political threat –
as one Conservative cabinet minister complained in the 1990s, 'decent'
people have to step over them on the way out of the opera. The overwhelming struggle simply for day-to-day survival leaves little time or
energy for political mobilisation and action, and the problems they
pose have usually been dealt with through a limited range of responses
from studious neglect to outright repression. What preoccupied social

reformers at the end of the nineteenth century was the fear that their ranks would, as a result of widespread unemployment, be joined by those with greater experience of organisation and activism. This problem was compounded by the fact that the state's response to unemployment and poverty was limited to a singular repressive and deterrent Poor Law which was incapable of discriminating between the two. It was in this context that social investigators and reformers were to push for a new conceptualisation and definition of poverty in which the 'poor' were to be redefined as a minority of the working class and poverty re-cast, not as a condition of those forced to earn a living, but as the lack of a certain minimum level of income. In so doing, a wedge was to be driven between the poor and the poorest. The necessity for this distinction was succinctly expressed by Charles Booth:

> The question of those who actually suffer from poverty should be considered separately from that of the true working classes, whose desire for a larger share of the wealth is of a different character. It is the plan of the agitators and the way of sensational writers to confound the two in one . . . . .To confound these essentially distinct problems is to make the solution of both impossible.
>
> (Booth 1904: 155)

Some way had therefore to be found of establishing new forms of relief, restricted to the 'deserving' unemployed, that would mark out their separation. During the closing decades of the nineteenth century various schemes were tried out based largely on the provision of relief work, rather than the workhouse test. As the Conservative Prime Minister Arthur Balfour told the Royal Commission on the Poor Laws:

> We distinctly proposed to deal with the elite of the unemployed . . . The unemployed for whom the Bill was intended were respectable workmen settled in a locality, hitherto accustomed to regular work, but temporarily out of employment through circumstances beyond their control.
>
> (*Report of the Royal Commission on the Poor Laws and Relief of Distress* 1909, Vol. 1: 493)

Such measures would, it was hoped, not only remove the deserving unemployed from their association with the residuum, but also allow the much-discredited Poor Law to retain its punitive role. Joseph Chamberlain, who as President of the Local Government Board had initiated the first of these schemes immediately after the 1886 riots, explained his intentions in a private letter to Beatrice Webb:

> It will remove one great danger, viz. that public sentiment should go wholly over to the unemployed, and render impossible that state sternness to which you and I equally attach much importance . . . By offering reasonable work at low wages we may secure the power of being very strict with the loafer and the confirmed pauper.
>
> (cited Harris 1972: 76)

The various attempts to establish a system of relief works for the deserving unemployed proved ultimately unsuccessful, submerged beneath the large bureaucracy and heavy administrative costs of sifting through and assessing applicants to determine who would and who would not be eligible. By 1911, however, a more permanent solution was found. Drawing on the experience in Germany of Bismarck, 'who dealt the heaviest blow against German socialism', according to one reformer, 'not by his laws of oppression . . . but by that great system of state insurance which now safeguards the German worker at almost every point of his industrial career' (cited Gilbert 1966: 257), the introduction of a scheme of National Insurance for both sickness and unemployment benefit was to be the crowning act of a series of reforms. With benefits payable only to those who had made regular and continuous contributions, the scheme would, according to the civil servant responsible for drafting the legislation, 'automatically exclude the loafer' (Llewellyn-Smith 1910: 527) without the need for detailed personal investigation. Although rates of benefit were to be kept low so as to 'imply a sensible and even severe difference between being in work and out of work' (cited Harris 1972: 365), National Insurance was to provide benefits to the 'deserving' sick and unemployed as a matter of right. Its symbolism was captured by Winston Churchill in introducing the Bill to the House of Commons:

> The idea is to increase the stability of our institutions by giving the mass of industrial workers a direct interest in maintaining them. With a 'stake in the country' in the form of insurance against evil days these workers will pay no attention to the vague promises of revolutionary socialism . . . It will make him a better citizen, a more efficient worker, and a happier man.
>
> (cited ibid.)

## Social democracy

'The peculiar character of the social democracy', wrote Marx (1968: 121), 'is epitomised in the fact that democratic-republic institutions are demanded as a means, not of doing away with two extremes, capital and wage labour, but of weakening their antagonism and transforming it into harmony.' Certainly, the reforms of the Liberal government at the beginning of the twentieth century did not go so far as to demand the abolition of the monarchy or the creation of a republic in Britain, although they were to bring it into serious conflict with the House of Lords and, as a result, lead to a substantial reduction in the political power of the landed aristocracy. Nevertheless, the reform of social policy did represent a fundamental shift, and in both institutional and ideological terms established the foundation for the social-democratic 'welfare' state that was developed after the second world war. Although it is the post-war Labour government of 1945 that is conventionally credited with the creation of this welfare state, both its institutional forms (National Insurance, tripartism, an active state) and its ideological underpinnings (the rights of citizenship) were by then already well established.

The origins of Liberal social reform lay firmly within the ruling class. 'The present movement for social reform', noted one Liberal supporter, 'springs from above rather than from below . . . [It] is less the spontaneous demand of the working classes than the tactical inducement of the political strategist' (Atherley-Jones 1893: 629). For many of the working class social reform was, and for many still remains, at best a poor substitute for justice and equality, and at worst a guise for continued abuse. As Henry Pelling has argued,

> The extension of the power of the state at the beginning of this century which is generally regarded as having laid the basis of the welfare state was by no means welcomed by the working class, was indeed undertaken over the critical hostility of many of them, perhaps of most of them.
>
> (Pelling 1968: 2)

Central to this critique was the recognition that reform was intended to placate opposition and stave off more fundamental change. The Conservative MP Quintin Hogg saw this equally clearly in 1945: 'If you do not give the people social reform', he warned, 'they are going to give you social revolution' (cited Harris 1961: 5). Of course, from the point of view of the poor, the constant dilemma has been that social reform offers the possibility of some immediate benefit, however partial or limited this might be, while revolution is for the most part a distant and hazardous objective. At the beginning of the twentieth century this dilemma was the subject of considerable debate within the British labour movement. The annual report of Liverpool Trades Council for 1894, for example, noted how

> most of the Council didn't like it at all . . . But when we saw the starvation and misery existing in our midst through lack of employment we considered it our duty to help and find some method of easing the suffering of our contemporaries.
>
> (cited Thane 1984: 886)

Others were less ready to accept the bribes on offer, although their refusal to do so has frequently brought them criticism and ridicule. In 1944 Barbara Wootton continued this argument:

> Somebody on the left is sure to be saying that the Beveridge Report is only tinkering with the problem, and that we should not be distracted by trivial piecemeal reform, but should concentrate all our energies on 'getting socialism first' . . . The Beveridge plan is there, ready to go on the statute book as it stands. I suggest no one has the right to turn his back on it, in order to get socialism first, unless he has a plan for socialism which is equally ready to go into law at once – equally concrete, precise and detailed.
>
> (Wootton 1944: 12)

Beneath working-class scepticism about social reform, however, lay a much more fundamental distrust of the state that the experiment in social democracy attempted to overcome. Although from the beginning of the nineteenth century various individuals and organisations had developed theories of the class nature of the state, to a very considerable extent this distrust was based on a more generalised and common working-class experience. For most of its history this experience was of the state as a repressive institution: of a legislature which, until 1867, was exclusively in the control of property-owners, and which, even when the franchise began to be extended, would take a further fifty years to give a vote to the majority of working people; of a militia, a police force and an army which not infrequently was called upon to protect the interests of the rich and powerful, and of a Poor Law which treated the poor as criminals. For the most part the identity of the state was unambiguous: a player in the deeply divided class relationships that characterise British society. Richard Hoggart has described it like this:

> When I look back on my childhood in Hunslet, a working class district in Leeds, the aspects which have a special bearing on present changes are these. Firstly, a quite deeply rooted sense that we are at the thin end of society . . . that we lived in the grimy south of the town, on the wrong side of the river. On the other side there was a rather shadowy impalpable 'them': local authorities, Rating Officers, Public Assistance Officers, Welfare Officers . . . There was this initial imaginative division between us . . . We knew in our bones that this separation existed . . . As a kind of reaction to this there was also a quite tight sense of being a local neighbourhood; a sense of belonging to an area and a group. Much of this sense was defensive, obviously, but when you look at it closely, you see that it was not merely defensive. What impresses, I think more than anything, is the virtues it sustained . . . the creation of co-operatives and friendly societies . . . the interweaving of Christianity, socialism, a traditional 'peasant' community sense, a defensiveness against the bosses . . . all these things came together in one texture.
>
> (Hoggart 1960: 13)

Defensiveness can also become a form of opposition. The co-operatives and friendly societies, still present in the twentieth century, had during the nineteenth century been developed precisely against working-class experience of capitalism and state policy, providing goods and services, benefits and mutual aid through institutions that remained within working-class control. It was through such institutions that a collective sense of identity – of 'us' against 'them' – was nurtured and developed, and their very existence posed the possibility of an alternative social order. When, by the end of the nineteenth century, an explicitly socialist, and sometimes revolutionary, ideology was added, the challenge to the existing political establishment became clear. When even apologists for capitalism recognised its inability to maintain adequate levels of employment or prevent the growth of poverty and misery, the political consequences of working-class distrust threatened to become explosive.

It was in this context that social reform was to attempt to do more than offer concessions to the 'deserving' poor. The reforms of social democracy were to attempt to redefine the image of the state, 'to cultivate the conception', argued one reformer, 'that the state is not merely a necessary but a beneficent institution' (cited Corrigan 1977: 386). Or as Sidney Webb would have it:

> It seems desirable to promote in every way the feeling that 'the Government' is no entity outside of ourselves, but merely ourselves organised for collective purposes, regarding the state as a vast benefit society, of which the whole body of citizens are necessarily members.
>
> (Webb 1890: 104)

It was the recognition of this political necessity that was ultimately to distinguish the Fabian Society from the Charity Organisation Society, whose principled opposition to state intervention was to leave it out in the cold. But it was the Liberal government that was to put it into practice. This, according to Winston Churchill, was 'the great mission of Liberalism . . . to bring the people into government . . . to associate ever larger numbers with offices of authority' (cited Churchill 1967: 308).

The extension of parliamentary democracy and the right to vote, as with the other rights of citizenship, has been a carefully timed and orchestrated process (Corrigan and Sayer 1985; Saville 1957). In this the self-serving cynicism of the British ruling class, like its arrogance, knows no bounds. In 1872, in a passage that might have served as a salutary warning to Margaret Thatcher some 100 years later, the magazine *Vanity Fair* reflected on the granting of the franchise to skilled male workers some five years earlier:

> What will be the result of giving real power to the people of England no man can yet say, simply because no man has yet taken the trouble to understand the people of England. How should anybody? They live somewhere down in the East End among the docks, in rows of cottages in Manchester, and in shanties about the fields outside people's parks . . . It is impossible to make the acquaintance of creatures who don't go to dinner parties, and if we really have delivered ourselves into their hands let us simply hope for the best. At the worst we shall have to enlarge the workhouses. But it will be interesting to see what these creatures make of us their masters, and whether they intend to go on sending in supplies of grocers to play at being in politics and society. There is nothing so hateful as the Grocer, and the working man is far more intelligent, more honourable, more of a gentleman altogether – and, of course, we shall manage him just as we have always managed the grocers ever since we let them in.
>
> (cited McGregor 1957: 35)

So it was to prove, although the calculations were to be more difficult, the risks more uncertain, the political difficulties more fraught, and the resistance of the establishment to the necessity of reform more concerted than such an account suggests. It was, however, a task made easier by the decision of the trade-union movement to establish a political wing – later constituted as the Labour Party – to press in Parliament for the repeal of anti-union legislation. 'We heartily welcome the new Labour Party', argued the *Independent Review*, the magazine of the growing radical wing of the 'new' liberalism:

> It will be a gain to the cause of social reform, since no pressure from within the Liberal Party could prove so strong . . . We cannot suppress a smile when noticing the alarm caused in a section of our press by the victory of the workers. The latter are asserting that the rich are now confronted with grave peril . . . We hold a different opinion. Probably no less than twenty three of the twenty nine new M.P.s will call themselves socialists. But their socialism is rather an ideal, a point of view, than a programme of action . . . As far as we can see at present, we are convinced that we shall never have occasion to differ.
>
> (cited Rothstein 1929: 289)

Such faith was to be repaid by the first leader of the Labour Party, Ramsay MacDonald, whose view was that the Labour Party would 'never willingly touch a slum population', and whose vision of Labour politics was based not on 'a process of economic reasoning, or of working class experience [but] upon conceptions of right and wrong common to all classes' (cited Rothstein 1929: 290). In 1931 MacDonald abandoned the Labour Party to join with Liberals and Conservatives in the formation of a National Government prepared to push through cuts in unemployment benefit during the second great depression. But while the Labour Party, like all parties, has had its share of traitors, the far greater tragedy has been the tireless effort, sacrifice and dedication of thousands of Labour Party members and supporters, beguiled by the lure of parliamentary democracy into thinking that capitalism could be tamed, or that capital would ever allow them to breach the bastions of privilege and power.

While the 'new' liberalism was to embrace the Labour Party, it was also to attempt to incorporate other working-class institutions, most notably the trade-union movement and the vast network of working-class friendly societies, who were to be given seats on advisory committees for the new institution of Labour Exchanges and in the administration of the National Insurance scheme: a tactic intended, according to Winston Churchill, to 'so far demonstrate the complexity of the problem as to dispose finally of all rough and ready revolutionary solutions' (cited Harris 1972: 365). Such a move was of course fraught with difficulty. In general, the organisation of workers is anathema to capital, as the attacks on trade unionism in recent years have demonstrated, but just as capital was willing to countenance the involvement of 'responsible' trade unionism in the tripartite arrangements that characterised the welfare settlement after the second world war, so too political realism in the early twentieth century demanded a radical accommodation. This was one which would also draw a distinction between the trade-union leadership and its rank-and-file organisation. As the Liberal Party newspaper argued in support of the engineering workers' union in their dispute with employers in 1897:

> Trades unionism is a force which on the whole makes for rational conservatism. It gives responsibility to those men who are marked out as the natural leaders of democracy. It is a school of government. It is certainly a barrier against the more formless and ill-considered kinds of socialist theory.
>
> (cited Rothstein 1929: 272)

But perhaps the most lasting legacy of the 'new' liberalism, and its contribution to the social democratic project, was its elaboration of entitlement to welfare as a mark of citizenship. As a concept, citizenship offered membership of, rather than exclusion from, the political body, but it is also an individualising concept: it offers this to people as individuals rather than as members of collectivities. It is also something that can be denied to other individuals. Thus National Insurance – and the inclusion of 'nation' in its title reflected this – would offer benefits as a right of citizenship without the stigma of the Poor Law to some, while others would remain excluded from it. Significantly, those excluded and forced to claim poor relief also lost the right to vote. Llewellyn-Smith encapsulated this dual strategy of adjustment to the growing political power of the working class, while maintaining a punitive policy towards its poorest members: 'military discipline', he argued, 'is right for the submerged; but democracy is the only hope for labour in general' (cited Davidson 1971: 227).

The elaboration of new forms of social policy, and of a new more active role for the state, was one thing; persuading employers and the rest of the ruling class to accept this, and to pay for it, was another.

'What we have to do is to detach the great employer', argued Beatrice Webb, 'whose profits are too large to feel the pressure of regulation and who stands to gain by the increased efficiency of the factors of production, from the ruck of small employers or stupid ones. What seems clear is that we shall get no further instalments of social reform unless we gain the consent of an influential minority of the threatened interest' (cited Saville 1957: 9).

Capital is not an homogeneous entity; its division in different parts of the economy – finance, trade, manufacturing, etc. – and the division within these between large and small enterprises, each with their differing interests, makes concerted action on the part of capital difficult. Although the purpose of capital in general is to increase surplus value, and to enrich itself, the different factions have differing interests, differing ways of doing this, as well as differing degrees of power. This was particularly well illustrated in the debates about labour conditions at the beginning of the twentieth century: the existence of a sizeable group of small employers, able to compete with their larger counterparts only by driving down wages and working conditions, was seen as contributing to the decline in national efficiency and to growing social unrest. In the 'national interest' – that is, in the interest of the long-term viability of capitalism as a whole – their activities would have to be curbed. The extreme reluctance to broach the principle that the state should not interfere with private property meant that the extent of regulation was very limited, but the 1906 Wages Act, introducing minimum wages into certain of the 'sweated industries', marked a significant step in the state's role. The abolition of this legislation by the Thatcher government equally marked the changed political context of the late twentieth century.

The task of the state, at least as identified by social reformers at the beginning of the twentieth century, was not only to curb the socially and economically damaging excesses of sweat-shop capitalism; it was also to identify, and where necessary organise, the interests of capital as a whole. Capital, both large and small, thrives on competition, but this also prevents it from taking those costly steps which are economically or politically necessary for fear of being undercut by its rivals. Only the state is capable of resolving this dilemma, by forcing all to fall into line. But first they had to be persuaded of the necessity of reform, and of their own interest in paying something for it. In part, therefore, social reformers were to appeal to the economic self-interest of employers: 'Money which is spent on maintaining the health, the vigour, the efficiency of mind and body in our workers', argued Lloyd George in pressing his scheme for National Health Insurance, 'is the best investment in the market' (Lloyd George 1911: 781), and all employers would be expected to pay their share. As he further argued in the *Times*:

> German experience shows that organised provision for the health of the working classes produces increased efficiency. I have no doubt that a similar result will be experienced when the demoralising anxieties of unemployment are mitigated. If, as I hope, these influences more than counterbalance the burden we are asking employers to bear, the cost of production will be diminished rather than increased.
>
> (*Times* 12 May 1911)

It remained, however, a testament to the strength of the vile maxim that even appeals to long-term economic self-interest frequently fell on deaf ears. A short-term pursuit of profit and reluctance to invest in the future has characterised British capitalism throughout its history. If capital was to be persuaded of the need to pay for social reform, then it would have to be frightened into doing so. 'We should boldly take our stand on the facts', argued Haldane, 'and proclaim the policy of taking, mainly by direct taxation, such toll from the increase and growth of wealth as will enable us to provide for the increasing cost of social reform . . . The more boldly such a proposition is put the more attractive I think it will prove. It will commend itself to many timid people as a bulwark against the Nationalisation of Wealth' (cited Harris 1972: 270).

It was in this role that the radical edge and language of the 'new' liberalism was decisive: Lloyd George, its most prominent spokesman, appealed directly to the working class, berating the short-sightedness of the ruling class and engineering a populist pressure for reform. He was, according to Lenin, 'a first class bourgeois businessman and master of political cunning, a popular orator, able to make any kind of speech, even revolutionary speeches, before labour audiences . . . Lloyd George serves the bourgeoisie splendidly' (cited Adams 1953: 64).

The extension of the power of the state at the beginning of the twentieth century, and its limitations on the unfettered freedom of private property to do whatever it liked, were intended to secure the long-term interests and stability of capitalism against the challenges it faced. In doing so the state established the framework of social democracy that would be significantly expanded in the three decades following the second world war. That these earlier reforms, like those that would follow later, were carried out often in the name of socialism merely reflected the widespread use, and abuse, of the term, and the differing purposes to which it could be put. For as one commentator noted in 1888:

> We are all socialists in the sense that our aim is the improvement of society. But there are socialists and Socialists . . . The socialists with a big 'S' have proved immensely serviceable to the more rational body of reformers by forcing inquiry upon sluggish minds.
>
> (Arnold 1888: 560)

The hijacking of the term socialism to serve the interests of capitalism did not however challenge the fundamental purposes of state policy:

> If we are all socialists now, as is so often said, it is not because we have undergone any change of principles of social legislation, but only a public awakening to our social miseries . . . We are all socialists now, only in feeling as much interest in these grievances as the Socialists are in the habit of doing, but we have not departed from our old lines of social policy.
>
> (Rae 1890: 439)

## The welfare state

These old lines of social policy were to be continued in the construction of the welfare state after 1945. In many cases these reforms had already been decided upon, and owed little to the Labour government with which they have conventionally been associated. The 1943 Education Act, for example, was itself the work of the Conservative war-time Education Minister Rab Butler, while according to Sir John Walley, formerly Deputy Secretary in the Ministry of Pensions and National Insurance, 'the basic ideas of the Beveridge Report could hardly have surprised anyone versed in current thinking about social security in the 1920s' (Walley 1972: 40). Beveridge himself was similarly aware of his own proposals' historical pedigree: 'The scheme proposed here is in some ways a revolution, but in more important ways it is a natural development from the past. It is a British revolution' (Beveridge 1942: 31). It was the rhetoric – of state provision for citizens 'from the cradle to the grave', of equality of opportunity, the abolition of the 'five giants' of disease, ignorance, squalor, idleness and want – rather than the reality of change within the welfare state which figured most prominently. Certainly there were innovations, of which the National Health Service was the most distinctive. The state's commitment to maintain full employment, while well rehearsed by Keynes in the 1930s, was also something new, although it is questionable how far this commitment was put to the test. The long boom which followed post-war reconstruction saw unemployment remain well below what state planners had envisaged as economically possible, and it was this rather than the welfare state which provided the basis for steadily increasing, although still unequal, standards of living.

Beneath the rhetoric, the old lines of social policy, if not immediately visible, continued to work their way. The post-war welfare settlement continued to favour white male skilled workers, confirming the priorities set for social policy in support of the labour market. Women, the working-class elderly, sick and disabled, as the 'rediscovery' of poverty in the 1960s confirmed, appeared low down the list of priorities. Newcomers too to Britain, or at least those with black faces who were recruited to fill the gaps in low-paid work created by the boom, although British citizens in name, found that their citizenship was distinctly second-class (Harris 1991).

But if the rhetoric of welfare was stronger than its reality, rhetoric also had its consequences. If the rhetoric of the welfare state stressed equality of opportunity and the rights of citizens, it could not easily prevent those citizens from demanding their opportunities and rights. From the 1960s onwards, inspired by the example of the civil-rights and black-power movements in the USA, a ferment of political protest embracing black people, the women's movement, gays and lesbians, the disabled and the poor was to grow and, critically, to demand of the state that it deliver on its pledges. Despite attempts to ignore these demands, or where they could not be ignored to minimise their impact, welfare spending and welfare activity grew.

Had the working class accepted the post-war settlement of 1945, and demanded no more, then it is possible that the welfare state would have had a longer existence. But history does not stand still. Neither does capital. Its unprecedented expansion during the post-war boom began by the 1970s to falter. The drive to maintain profit levels was to accelerate its expansion, in search of cheaper labour and bigger markets. Domestically it led to a questioning of the cost that the post-war settlement had imposed. It is arguable whether the greater 'cost' was economic – the welfare state after all resulted only in a relatively slight redistribution of income and wealth – or political. Either way, the settlement was not to be maintained, and in its breaking capital was decisively to claw back many of the gains that the poor had made.

## The neo-liberal project

The neo-liberal project that set itself to transform economic and social relationships in Britain and elsewhere aimed no less than to break the post-war settlement and to transfer the balance of economic, social and political power decisively in favour of capital and its allies. Centrally this was to involve a reassertion of the authority of employers over workers in the workplace. But this in turn was to depend upon a dismantling of the rights and securities afforded to people by the welfare state and full employment, and a reversal of the movement towards greater equality and the popular expectations and political aspirations that had accompanied the post-war boom. The new right which emerged from the political wilderness during the course of the 1970s was to give this project its political leadership.

The rise of the new right is a political success story of the first order, akin to the triumph of bourgeois political economy – the 'old' liberalism of the early nineteenth century which it largely emulated – or the 'new' liberalism and social democracy which it sought to replace. That it was able to gain widespread support for the ideas it represented – the superiority of the unfettered market, the need to reduce the power of the state – ideas which had been on the fringes of the political establishment since at least the second world war, is testament to its powers of organisation as much as to its political opportunism. The new right's appeal was to those who felt threatened and disillusioned, and there were many of these. They ranged from rich to poor, who either thought their wealth was threatened or who wanted the opportunity to gain a greater share, from racists and bigots to those who found the changing world of 'race' and gender unsettling and confusing, and to whom the appeal to 'traditional' values of respect for authority, order and the patriarchal family offered some stability and comfort. It even appealed to the poorest, who would suffer the most from its depredations, for whom the state had provided little, and whose experience of its petty rules and regulations framed a ready support for promises to 'get the state off our backs'.

In their various organisational settings radical conservatives who had become increasingly alarmed by the consequences of social democracy launched a remarkable counter-offensive in which they weaved together cultural, social, political and economic developments and events to present a world view of capitalism in dire crisis. In this, explanations for the faltering of the post-war boom and the threat of its imminent collapse were to be sought, not in the dynamics of the capitalist economy itself, but in the growth of a welfare state and its social and cultural consequences. What many had considered to be signs of progress – women's rights, civil rights, greater sexual freedom, an active state welfare policy (however flawed), cultural developments and active citizenship as people mobilised and took an interest in local and national politics – were all reconstructed as threats to capitalism and the free-enterprise society.

In the context of the USA, the Silks wrote:

> . . . after the long era of post-war good (or at least relatively good) feeling between business and labour, business and the intellectuals, business and the liberals, business and government, business and the blacks and other social groups, an era of business defensiveness mixed with hostility emerged in the 70s. This hostile mood of business was a response to these events: the Watergate scandals in which over 200 business corporations were involved through illegal campaign contributions; improper corporate payments abroad . . . Corporate executives felt put upon – by organised labour, liberals, blacks, environmentalists, women and other critical public interest groups and their lawyers, and perhaps most of all by the rise of new and costly forms of government regulation in such areas as occupational health and safety, air and water pollution and equal employment rules.
>
> Rather than accept such public criticism and regulation as a just and necessary corrective for wrong doing, businessmen generally regarded the attacks as exaggerated, unfair, a threat (deliberate or unconscious) to the very existence of the free enterprise system. Business suffered from an acute feeling that its enemies were closing in on it.
>
> (Silk and Silk 1980: 253)

The new right benefited enormously from this business anxiety both in the USA and Britain. For most of the post-war period far right radical conservatives had had little influence or power and saw themselves as 'the remnant' – 'a small, highly educated elite that kept alive the flames of truth and freedom in an age of encroaching darkness. They were critics of, rather than participants in, mass society and politics' (Judis 1983: 22). From the mid-1970s these remnants, organised in small think tanks such as the Institute of Economic Affairs in the UK and the Heritage Foundation and American Enterprise Institute (AEI) in the USA, saw a dramatic change in their fortunes as corporate funds flowed in their direction. The Heritage Foundation (founded in 1973 and launched with a grant of $250,000 from the anti-union brewer Joseph Coors) saw its income rise to $2,116,448 by 1977 and to $8,617,977 in 1982. The AEI similarly saw its budget increase from $1 million in 1971 to over $10 million by 1981. As the *New York Times Magazine* (10 May 1982: 65), observed, the AEI 'has connected with a new consciousness and mood in the business community that emphasises the importance of funding research and writing that will help further the views of American corporations and the shape of public policy accordingly'.

This flow of corporate funding transformed the fortunes of the new right. No longer remnants, they flourished in new think tanks (such as the Adam Smith Institute in London) and established themselves in a position to generate ideas and reports on key elements of a new social, economic and political agenda. With formal and informal links, the think tanks formed a new transatlantic alliance which prospered in the Reagan/Thatcher years. Staff were exchanged, ideas pooled, and a significant ideological base was formed to service the new conservative governments in both America and Britain. It was from these think tanks that both administrations drew their main intellectual support and in whose seminars and conferences ministers and officials sounded out their ideas and plans. They provided a key alternative to the established political and civil-service structures of the social-democratic state that the new right inherited but deeply distrusted.

The new right's success was largely predicated on its capacity to offer specific policy prescriptions which resonated with global capitalism's anxiety about the limitations and threats emanating from the social-democratic arrangements that had been secured in the leading capitalist societies. These anxieties find their most clear expression in the deliberations of the Trilateral Commission, formed in 1973 'by private citizens of Western Europe, Japan and North America to foster closer co-operation among those three regions on common problems' (Trilateral Commission 1979: front cover). Comprising members from

> most of the major Western and Japanese banks, corporations, senior law firms, former diplomats, bureaucrats and politicians, media proprietors and editors and 'policy oriented academics', along with a sprinkling of trade unionists . . . the Trilateral Commission is a mechanism for lubricating the thrust of co-operation and co-ordination between the major capitalist economies.
> (Gill 1980: 39–40)

In many respects it sets out the broad parameters of what came to be the new right's agenda.

As Gill points out, it is possible to over-estimate the importance of the Commission. Given the differences within global capitalism, it can be very difficult to arrive at trilateral solutions in areas such as economic and energy policies. However, the Commission's 1975 report entitled *The Crisis of Democracy* (Crozier et al. 1975) was of great importance in setting out elite opinion on the crisis of the state and identifying key policy targets which over the next twenty-five years were pursued with fanatical vigour in both the USA and Britain.

The three sociologists who were appointed to compile the report – Michael Crozier, Samuel Huntington and Joji Watanuki – identified what they saw as a fundamental 'paradox' at the heart of social democracy. This was that the increase in material prosperity of the 1950s and 1960s had been accompanied by an increase rather than a reduction in social tension (evidenced, for example, in the black-power, civil-rights and women's movements, and in anti-war and student protests). Their explanation was that:

> As happens everywhere, change produces rising expectations which cannot be met by its necessarily limited outcomes. Once people know that things can change, they cannot accept easily any more the basic features of their condition that were once taken for granted.
>
> (Crozier et al. 1975: 22)

The result was that:

> Previously passive or unorganised groups in the population, blacks, Indians, Chicanos, white ethnic groups, students and women now embarked on concerted efforts to establish their claims to opportunities, positions and rewards and privileges to which they had not previously considered themselves entitled.
>
> (Crozier et al. 1975: 61-2)

This in turn was to put increasing pressure on the state, overloading its capacities, while its unwillingness or inability to respond fed further discontent and a questioning of its authority and legitimacy. The result was 'the disintegration of civil society, the breakdown of social discipline, the debility of leaders and the alienation of citizens' (Crozier et al. 1975: 2).

Arguing that 'some of the problems of governance in the United States today stem from an excess of democracy', Huntington in his US section of the report concluded that what was 'needed instead is a greater degree of moderation in democracy' (cited Sklar (ed.) 1980:

37). Crozier, who wrote the European section, was no less pessimistic about the so-called 'democratic surge' and the challenge this posed to government as 'democratic societies cannot work when the citizenry is not passive' (Wolfe 1980: 298). Thus the stage was to be set for an attempt to reduce popular expectations and restructure and redefine the responsibilities of government.

The neo-liberal project, however, had also to confront what was seen as an additional cause of this crisis. According to the Trilateral report, the growth of social tensions had been fuelled by the activities of some 'intellectuals and related groups who assert their disgust with the corruption, materialism and inefficiency of democracy and with the subservience of democratic governments to "monopoly capitalism"' (cited ibid.). It identified in particular a stratum 'of value-oriented intellectuals who often devote themselves to the derogation of leadership, the challenging of authority, and the unmasking and delegitimation of established institutions' (cited Chomsky 1977: 10). These intellectuals – identified as the significant opinion-formers in society, but above all as welfare professionals: a 'new class' of social workers, psychologists, probation officers, school and university teachers amongst others – came to occupy a central place in the subsequent new-right critique. As both the product and the principal beneficiaries of the expanded social-democratic welfare state which placed such trust in 'experts' to bring about social improvement, the new class in its questioning and scepticism was held to be particularly responsible for the collapse in traditional authority and the 'lack of willingness to acclaim and obey' without question (Habermas 1983: 77). Above all they were seen to be opposed to the values of free enterprise and capitalism. According to Irvin Kristol, one of the most influential of new-right intellectuals: 'The simple truth is that the professional classes of our modern bureaucratised society are engaged in a class struggle with the business community for status and power. Inevitably this class struggle is conducted under the guise of "equality"' (*New York Times Magazine* 10 May 1982).

Thus the social-democratic welfare state was implicated at the heart of the crisis of capitalism: it had generated the layers of welfare professionals who were so 'disdainful' of old authority and questioned capitalism's capacity for social justice. It was state welfare that was held responsible for the 'explosion' of expectations and the demanding of rights on the part of the previously 'passive' groups of women, black people and the poor that led to the overloading of the state. It too was accused of providing the material means whereby working people could engage in industrial disputes and resist the demands of employers (Jones and Novak 1985), for as Bluestone and Harrison have argued:

> to make really significant, long-term dents in labour costs . . . workers would have to be made so insecure and desperate for work that they would be forced to become more 'flexible', that is, more willing to accept management's new terms with respect to wages, working conditions and discipline . . . The only way for capital to . . . produce the necessary amount of insecurity was to attack the social wage itself.
>
> (Bluestone and Harrison 1982: 180)

This assault on the social wage was also to require an assault on those who provided it and the ideologies which underpinned it. Berated as 'monopoly producers' who denied people 'freedom of choice', state welfare professionals were subjected to a populist critique in which the new right skilfully mobilised people's ambivalence towards state provision and its domination by bureaucrats and experts. At the same time it embarked upon a repudiation of equality as a legitimate goal of government or principle of social organisation. As Samuel Brittan wrote in 1976:

> The ideal of equality has had a noble role in human history. It has served to assert that all men and women are entitled to respect, and to rally people against oppression. But it has now turned sour. Liberal democracy will not be saved by detailed policy programmes which will soon be overtaken by events. It could yet be saved if contemporary egalitarianism were to lose its hold over the intelligentsia. But this will happen only if those who recognise it for the disease it has become are prepared to come out in the open.
>
> (Brittan 1976: 133)

By the 1980s the new right were not only out in the open, but firmly established in power; confident enough to declare, as did Kenneth Baker, Secretary of State for Education, when introducing his Education Reform Bill at the 1987 Conservative Party conference, that 'the pursuit of egalitarianism is now over'. History will tell if he spoke too soon, but that he spoke at all is testament to the transformation that has taken place.

# 5 Re-tooling the state

'I think we will have to go back to soup kitchens', she told him and paused. Then, noting his reaction, she continued, 'Take that silly smile off your face. I mean it.'

(Margaret Thatcher to Patrick Jenkin, Secretary of State for Social Services, April 1979, in Davies 1997: 287)

The welfare state that marked the lives of a generation in a number of advanced capitalist societies after the second world war now appears as a relatively brief interlude in the otherwise dismal role of state policy in its dealings with the poor. Its departure from the usual lines of business was, over time, to engage the state in an unprecedented range of organisation, provision and regulation of economic and social life. This was to have enormous implications, not only for people's standard of living but also for popular expectations and for a belief in the ability or at least the responsibility of government to do something about unemployment, inequality and poverty. In the process state policy became an increasingly contested area, and a focus for mobilisation and organisation of a diverse range of groups that were to push the state into its constantly expanding role.

The reasons for this expansion of state activity were varied, reflecting its accommodation to the disparate range of interests and pressures that formed the post-war settlement and its subsequent development. From the point of view of capital – the dominant partner to the settlement – a 'modern' national post-war economy required at least a basic infrastructure (a national system of banking, of communications and transport and of energy) which in many countries the state came to supply. Industry similarly had other demands: a minimal level of health, training and sometimes education amongst its workforce, or the organisation of the labour market, which in general it preferred to have funded at the public expense. The welfare state bore this imprint, focused on the maintenance and reproduction of breadwinners – especially male – to the relative neglect of the 'Cinderella' services that catered for the disabled, mentally ill and others whose labour was not in demand. (This in turn impacted differentially on women, leaving those who were unable to afford private care services to bear the brunt of care for many of their dependent relations and friends.) For capital the state was also to be an important organiser of economic demand – as employer, purchaser and redistributor of income – maintaining the buoyancy of consumption and production.

As a point of principle there was little new in this. Throughout its history, the development of capitalism and the development of the state have been coterminous. From the mercantilist state of the seventeenth and eighteenth centuries, through the supposed 'laissez-faire' state of the nineteenth, the power of the state was actively used to fashion the requirements of an expanding capitalism. Its significantly expanded role in the second half of the twentieth century was not without its critics and opposition, especially when, as in the protracted battles over the steel industry, it threatened to nationalise more profitable and lucrative concerns. But in the main, capital – and large-scale capital in particular – was content to accept the creation of an infrastructure of state policy in areas such as social security, health and education that would both meet the minimal requirements of productivity and social order and, most importantly, attempt to secure the social relationships and ideologies that justified enduring poverty and inequality.

If the state's expanded role as handmaiden of a profitable economy was accepted by capital, at least for a time, as an extended version of what had gone before, what gave the welfare state its distinctive characteristic was by and large the result of popular pressure. The search for a just society after the second world war was to give the welfare state its democratic appeal, and popular demands were to counter – with greater or lesser degrees of success – the naked expression of capital's demands. Questions such as what was to count as education, or whose interests welfare should serve, increasingly became areas of public debate. Significantly, it was those parts of the welfare state furthest removed from market principles that proved most popular, in particular the creation of a National Health Service based on need rather than ability to pay and embodying strong traditions of public service. But elsewhere the expansion of the welfare state also created the opportunity for the development of public space and the de-commodification of important areas of life. Throughout its short life these countervailing claims on welfare were repeatedly contested, and policy developed in a series of skirmishes that at different times and in different arenas advanced and retarded political struggle.

From the mid-1970s the expanded role of the state was to be challenged by the new right, and in significant respects thrown into reverse. This is not to say that the state ceased its interventionist role, although the style and purpose of its intervention were to change considerably, still less that it loosened its grip on the levers of political power. Indeed, and in Britain in particular, the call of the new right to 'roll back the state' was to disguise its increasing centralisation of state power.

The scale and extent of the changes imposed on British society under the neo-liberal onslaught were to be such as to provoke a crisis even within the state itself. Significant parts of the establishment were to become critics of government policy, if only for their concern over what many saw as the excesses of Thatcherism and the impact of increasing social division and its implications for social stability and order. The Church of England frequently crossed swords with the government over deepening poverty and inequality; scientists and scholars recoiled at its philistine attacks on education and research; the House of Lords on more than one occasion attempted to block its measures; and even the monarchy on occasion barely concealed a growing rift with the course of political events. In some cases this was to lead to their silencing and containment. The opposition of the mass of the people – as instanced in widespread support for the miners in their showdown confrontation with the state in 1984-5, at Greenham Common, or in the opposition to the Poll Tax that was finally to precipitate the unceremonious removal of 'the Iron Lady' from power – called for a more systematic response. The growth of the secret intelligence service and a greater use of state surveillance, an increasingly militarised police force, and a raft of legislation curbing the rights of citizens and increasing the judicial power of the state were some of the means used to silence opponents. 'Democratic' opposition, in the form of locally elected councils, were largely stripped of their powers, and what remained subjected to central financial and legislative control. Out of this has emerged a state whose authoritarian capabilities have been greatly enhanced.

## Getting the state out of politics

The neo-liberal critique of the state was, with the exception of the right-wing 'libertarian' fringe that argued for the complete removal of all state restrictions, not a critique of state activity in general. On the contrary, state power was perceived to have a legitimate role in the maintenance of law and order, in ensuring the untroubled operation of the market, and in buttressing what it saw as the weakened role of the 'traditional' patriarchal family and the declining values of moral order. What exercised the new right was what it saw as the state's illegitimate incursions into the market and its unwarranted restrictions on private property and capital. Above all its target was what it caricatured as 'the nanny state': the system of benefits, protective legislation and welfare services which, it argued, had feather-bedded the population, and the poor in particular, had undermined the family and the values of thrift, discipline and hard work, and had brought about economic, social, cultural and moral decline. The new right in effect was forcefully restating a classical conservative perspective on the state in which it was deemed legitimate for the state to be the handmaiden of the market but illegitimate as a welfare agency other than in the provision of a basic and circumscribed safety net for the most destitute.

Beneath this concern lay the fears identified by the new right in the 1970s for the increasing politicisation of state activity. As the Trilateral Commission had warned, the expanded role of the state, as employer and as provider of an increasing range of services, had not only fuelled popular expectations and demands but had drawn the state ever more into the role of arbiter of industrial disputes and manager of social conflict. It was this face of state activity that was to be rolled back, while its coercive edge was to be strengthened to enable it to do so and to deal with its consequences. The depoliticisation of state activity and the attempt to relieve it of the pressures of popular expectations and competing claims about how society should be organised and managed lay in a fundamental sense at the heart of the neo-liberal project. Thus the privatisation of state-controlled industries, of British Airways, coal, gas, electricity and water supplies to name but a few, while it boosted state finances and provided a massive windfall to those who bought shares at knock-down prices, in more important ways also served to divest the state of responsibility to the workers they employed or the consumers they supplied. In future the supposed unquestionable and unchallengeable rule of market forces would determine levels of employment and conditions of work, while those with a complaint would no longer have recourse to publicly accountable officials or government itself.

State provision of welfare services was similarly if not more so seen as engendering public dissatisfaction and fuelling rising demands. As the veteran right-wing politician Enoch Powell argued in 1972:

The translation of a want or need into a right is the most widespread and dangerous of modern heresies . . . It provides unlimited fuel for dissatisfaction; it provides unlimited scope for the fostering of animosities between one set of potential recipients and another . . . The result is that ever wider and deeper state intervention is demanded while the state itself becomes the source, as well as the focus, of social grievances.

(cited George and Wilding 1976: 12)

The removal of the state from welfare provision, and with that its removal as the focus of popular demands and expectations, was a more difficult proposition. In social security, and especially in provision for the poorest, as also in areas of health, education and other services, there was little evidence that the private market was willing or able to take on any except provision for the more affluent. The proposal in the 1986 Green Paper on the reform of social security to privatise the State Earnings Related Pension Scheme (SERPS), for example, fell when the private insurance industry dismissed the scheme as unworkable and financially unattractive. In the face of this SERPS was substantially modified and left to decline. While some services were successfully transferred to the private sector, such as the provision of sickness benefit or many of the activities of local government, other areas of state provision were to be starved of resources and their deterioration left as an incentive to those who could afford it to buy their health or education elsewhere.

That provision which remained in the hands of the state was to be transformed even further. Where the market could or would not provide, 'quasi-markets' were introduced to imitate its disciplines, while businessmen were appointed in the place of doctors or teachers to manage the health and education services. Public accountability was withdrawn and replaced by government-appointed and publicly unanswerable quangos that have come to dominate the administration of public services. Above all, the reining-in of state welfare provision has had at its heart the dismantling of the notion of rights and the structures of entitlement that fuelled the expansion of the post-war welfare state. Popular expectations of a right to housing, to education, to a decent standard of living, to security in poverty, sickness or old age, and the countless other rights demanded by the poor, by women, by black people and others that were seen by the new right as undermining the future of capitalism and the state itself have been removed. In their place has been left a system that is deeply conditional and restricted and whose coercive edge serves as a reminder of the limits of state responsibility.

## A necessary compromise

The disciplinary activities of the state have always been a part of its operation and have always been present in its activities. The state is an instrument of domination, and although the forms of this domination have changed, in what might generally be termed a shift from coercion to consent, elements of coercion have always underpinned its activities. In the final analysis, the welfare state was no exception, underpinned by a hard edge of coercion for those who did not conform – the iron fist in the velvet glove as it was commonly characterised by the left during the early 1970s. But since then the velvet glove has slipped, revealing ever more in its daily practices and policies the hard edge beneath.

The experience of the reappearance of a more authoritarian state has of course been differentiated. Not all have felt its steely edge, although few have escaped its seepage into general political, social and cultural life. The intolerance and authoritarianism that marked in particular the leadership of Margaret Thatcher, the growth of racism and xenophobia, and the growing demand for 'law and order' have left their mark on a society that is less at ease with itself than for many generations. But for the most part this authoritarianism has impacted most on the poorest. And amongst the poorest, black inner-city communities and women have been most affected. The political appeal of 'Middle England', with both main political parties vying to attract the votes of a relatively affluent, powerful but threatened and declining minority in order to gain or keep themselves in office, has meant that for them the state has retained more of a benign face.

In the early 1960s Richard Titmuss was one of the first to draw attention to the 'hidden' welfare state of public tax subsidies to the private and occupational welfare schemes enjoyed largely by the middle classes. Since then this extensive package of benefits to private home ownership, private and occupational pensions, and private health and education has grown significantly, although characteristically without the expressed concern for the demoralising effects on its recipients that surrounded direct state provision. Equally in their consumption of state welfare services, especially in health and in further and higher education, where they have taken the largest share, the interests of Middle England have tempered attempts to restrict availability or impose costs. In general the middle classes have done well out of state welfare. Even after two decades of retrenchment – a retrenchment less marked in those areas on which the middle classes depend than in those that cater exclusively for the poor – state welfare continues to provide at best a valuable contribution to their standard of living and means of advancement, and at worst a declining set of services and benefits on which they have been able to build their own additional provision.

This is not to say that there have not been problems and conflicts. The professional middle classes, especially those working within the state sector whom the new right identified as 'the new class' that would pose particular difficulties for the restructuring of the state, have at times been in direct conflict with government. Their taming as a political and social force has been one of the significant achievements of the neo-liberal project. At the same time the neo-liberal project was to bring the new right into conflict with significant sections of the state machinery itself.

## Taking on the mandarins

The Thatcherite revolution in government went to the heart of 'the inbred political establishment' who Sir John Hoskyns, political adviser to the Prime Minister, dismissed as having suffered a 'massive failure of intelligence and nerve' in failing to confront the legacy of the 1960s and 1970s (*Financial Times* 29 September 1983). The radical reorientation of politics and policy that this would require would over the course of the next decade see this political establishment challenged and substantially reformed.

In this the senior ranks of the civil service were given early attention. At its higher levels, many were in any case suspect: themselves implicated in the 'consensus politics' of the post-war era and the corrupting influence of its welfare state. With such 'unreliable' advisers, Thatcher turned to the appointment of her own advisers from outside Whitehall, and their links with the new-right think tanks, which now became a central part of government policy-making.

In the short term the Whitehall mandarins were substituted in important areas of policy formation. Most of the ideas of the Thatcher governments – for deregulation or privatisation – came from outside Whitehall, accompanied by the belief that the existing administration was incapable of formulating and carrying through the radical change demanded. The role and influence of right-wing think tanks increased enormously, providing government with an agenda and a set of policies that were used to over-rule and over-ride civil-service misgivings and objections. The process then began of reorganising the machinery of state. In 1979 the head of Marks and Spencer, Sir Derek Rayner, later made Lord Rayner for his contribution, was appointed to head the Cabinet Office Efficiency Unit with a brief to bring a transforming realism to the civil service. At the same time the government embarked upon a sustained campaign of criticism that would seriously undermine civil-service morale. The ill-disguised contempt of the Prime Minister towards those senior civil servants 'not on her side' became a hall-mark of her administration, despite the occasional praise, as Sir Ian Bancroft put it, 'forced out between clenched teeth in public' (*Financial Times* 2 December 1983). Permanent Secretary of the Civil Service Department until his resignation the day after the Prime Minister ordered its abolition, Bancroft despaired of the impact of government criticism of its own senior staff: 'surely something has gone far wrong with any undertaking whose staff find it necessary to be furtive, evasive or apologetic about their occupation' (ibid.). In such a climate, criticism of government policy was muted if not silenced. As another top civil servant, Sir Patrick Nairne, Permanent Secretary at the DHSS between 1975 and 1981, put it rather more diplomatically, 'the repeated political attacks . . . have discouraged senior civil servants from arguing against aspects of policy against which they might have reservations' (Nairne 1983: 243). By 1988 twenty-four out of the twenty-seven permanent secretaries in post in Whitehall when Margaret Thatcher first took office had either resigned or retired. 'She has', according to the Political Editor of the *Observer* at the time, 'replaced them with men who tend to do things the Thatcher way' (*Observer* 21 February 1988).

By 1988 the reorganisation of the administrative branches of the civil service was in full swing. With their numbers reduced by 130,000 people, the government began what it called its 'Next Steps' reform aimed to transfer one in eight civil servants into twelve separate and semi-autonomous agencies. These agencies, with their own separate management structures, were to transform the internal relations of the state bureaucracy, replacing a unified administration guided at least in principle by an ethos of public service with structures more familiar in the world of private business. As one account of its implementation in the largest of these, the Benefits Agency created in 1991, noted:

> Central to this has been the reorganisation of local offices so that a layer of staff are redefined as management, with responsibilities for the organisation of work, the budgeting of the office and the implementation of state policy. Managerial hierarchies have been recomposed, with the down-playing of unifying and co-ordinating roles and an emphasis on supervision and control.
>
> (Carter and Fairbrother 1995: 139)

The effects of this 'new managerialism', with its changed working practices and conditions of work and its emphasis on working within newly devolved budgets and securing savings, have impacted not only on the front-line workers of the state bureaucracies, but also through them on the public they serve.

At the same time the Next Steps agencies introduced a separation between the formulation of policy, which remained the responsibility of government and its ministers, and the implementation of policy, now the responsibility of managers and from which ministers could, when convenient, distance themselves. The treatment of prisoners, for example, or the way in which benefits are paid out were matters largely removed from public scrutiny and democratic accountability and driven by cost-cutting and increased 'efficiency'. As Robert Harris, political editor of the *Observer*, argued at the time,

> it heralds the most fundamental reform of the civil service this cen-
> tury . . . The old Victorian ideal of a unified civil service,
> responsible through Ministers to Parliament, will be dead . . . In the
> long run this could prove one of the most far-reaching of all the
> Thatcherite reforms. Once undertaken, such a dispersal of power –
> often into the private sector – will be difficult for any subsequent
> government to reverse.
>
> (*Observer* 21 February 1988)

By 1995, rather than the twelve originally envisaged, over 100 such separate agencies had been created, from the Child Support Agency to HM Prison Service, employing 80 per cent of civil-service personnel (*Observer* 19 February 1995).

## Public misery, private gain

The transfer of the administration of public policy into the hands of the private sector which these reforms in part envisaged has advanced considerably, both in Britain and the USA. In both countries the sheer scale of state operations is such that major corporations have lined themselves up to bid for contracts. In Texas, plans were announced in 1997 to put out the administration of its entire welfare system to private tender. This led to the formation of consortia headed by three competing firms – Andersen Consulting, the world's biggest consultancy firm, Lockheed Martin, the world's biggest defence contractor, and Electronic Data Systems (EDS) – to bid for a contract estimated at $2–3 billion over five years. Elsewhere states have been privatising the administration of welfare since the late 1980s: Lockheed alone collects more than $1 billion a year of child-support payments on behalf of government, some 10 per cent of payments nation-wide, and has taken over the running of employment and training programmes in Dallas. It has also created a new division, Welfare Reform Initiative, to seek further contracts. EDS similarly runs child-welfare programmes in Illinois and California, and processes Medicaid claims in twenty different states (*Economist* 25 January 1997). As the *Economist* pointed out, the move to privatise welfare services in Texas 'raises more intractable issues. Because the private contractor will administer all social programmes, it will have to act with the authority of the state. That could mean refusing benefits to some people' (ibid.). It is a development that is eagerly watched; as the *Texas Observer* reported: 'Across the country, those with any interest in social services are watching what happens in Texas, and expecting that as Texas goes with welfare, so goes the nation' (*Texas Observer* 14 March 1997).

In Britain the private sector has similarly moved swiftly to compete for contracts not only in the administration of government services, such as that for one of the world's largest computer systems within the Department of Social Security, but also in the delivery of government policy and the direct provision of services. Private-sector provision and management of prisons, initiated by the Conservative government and denounced by the Labour Party in opposition as 'morally repugnant', is now accepted as government policy, attracting the attention of firms such as Securicor and the Correction Corporation of America. According to Alan Travis, within 'three years one in ten inmates will be in private jails in England and Wales, making ours one of the largest commercial penal industries in the world' (*Guardian* 26 August 1998). The insurance industry has similarly lined itself up to take advantage of those parts of the welfare system that offer commercial opportunities. In a document entitled 'The Transfer of Responsibility From the Public to the Private Sector' the Association of British Insurers made out its case to 'assist in any re-definition of the welfare state' and respond to 'opportunities which may arise' (cited *Guardian* 22 October 1993). Elsewhere the Private Finance Initiative has given private industry an expanded role in the building of schools, hospitals and public highways, while even the Department of Social Security has turned to selling off its debts to private debt-collecting agencies (*Guardian* 14 September 1995).

On an even greater scale legislation has forced the public sector to transfer provision and services to the private sector. The 1990 National Health Service and Community Care Act, for example, required local-authority social-services departments to put 85 per cent of their care budgets, such as for old people's or children's homes, out to the private market or voluntary sector, leaving the departments as purchasers and managers rather than providers of care for vulnerable people. The consequence, according to one local-authority social worker, is a system that is less accountable and more unstable:

> If it 'blows' in a voluntary sector organisation or a privately run home, they won't put up with it. They simply say 'Their bags are packed; come and take them.' Then we get someone back who's even more damaged than they started off being.
>
> (cited Novak and Sennett 1996: 75)

As for the voluntary sector, once noted for its independence and its ability to offer alternatives to the narrow confines of state policy, the lure of securing government contracts has led to a process of increasing competition and of adaptation to the 'contract culture', in which the purchasers retain the upper hand. This is how the manager of one voluntary organisation saw its new role:

> it has to sell itself: it has to do deals with local authorities, and the whole purchasing–providing split, as it's called, is not much of a split: you set out what your services are, and I guess you put the screws down on the cost of it.
>
> (ibid.)

This dispersal of state activity, whether to the voluntary sector, the private market or new semi-public agencies, is, as Clarke and Newman have pointed out, not a sign of its fragmentation or weakening:

> It may be more useful to describe these movements as dispersal rather than fragmentation. The concept of dispersal signals such processes as the effects of strategic calculation rather than inevitable occurrences . . . The state delegates – through a variety of means – its authority to subaltern organisations that thus are empowered to act on its behalf.
>
> (Clarke and Newman 1997: 25)

In this process the power of the state is extended, even where dispersal of responsibility for welfare is extended to the supposed private realm of the family. Thus the policy of community care, effectively of care for the elderly, sick or disabled by women in their families, represents

more than a shift towards expanded roles for the family and

reduced responsibilities for the state. The redrawing of the public/private distinction in the 1980s and 1990s has also produced greater state involvement in the private domain. The shift of responsibilities to families has been accompanied by the subjection of households to greater state surveillance, regulation and intervention. For example, the Child Support Agency, while being rhetorically defined as making parents 'responsible', has also created an apparatus of investigation and regulation. The 'criminalisation' of parents of delinquent children through the 1991 Criminal Justice Act has subjected familial relations to judicial intervention. The integration of 'primary carers' into the organisation of community care is not just a transfer of tasks and responsibilities to the private realm of the family. It also brings carers and their household arrangements into the realm of state assessment, evaluation and surveillance.

(Clarke and Newman 1997: 28–9)

This greater disciplinary involvement of the state in the private domain of working-class family life is set for further expansion in a number of policy areas. Clear examples are provided by the Parenting Orders and Child Safety Orders (child curfews) introduced under the New Labour government's 1998 Crime and Disorder Act. Both of these provisions place new legal obligations on parents to control their children, with criminal penalties for those who 'without reasonable excuse' have failed to address 'their child's anti-social or offending behaviour' (Home Office 1998: 5–6). As Goldson argues, these provisions are

predicated upon a pathologising and deeply offensive notion that parents of children in trouble 'wilfully refuse to accept their responsibilities' and negate the harsh material contexts invariably endured by such parents and their children. Two decades' worth of antagonistic social and economic policies have stripped resources and services from families with the greatest need for them . . . It is within this context that the Parenting Order is to impose – by way of criminal law – utterly unrealistic expectations on parents.

(Goldson 1999: 13)

These developments, whereby the state withdraws from the provision of services and resources but expands in ever more direct disciplinary ways into the once private domain of family life, are virtually without exception class-specific. It won't be the families of 'Middle England' who feel the weight of these laws but those living in the most hard-pressed regions of the country, including inner-city black populations who have long been seen by the state as criminogenic and in need of constant surveillance (Gutzmore 1983: 26).

## Unaccountable bodies

Alongside the reorganisation of the civil service and the machinery of state administration successive Conservative governments moved to quash potential opposition in the form of local authorities. As the major democratically elected alternative power base to central government, local councils were a constant thorn in the flesh of the new right's strategy to restructure welfare. The major providers of education, housing and personal social services, local authorities, increasingly elected during the 1980s to Labour Party control, struggled to deal with the devastating consequences of poverty and government policy on local communities. In some cases, as in Sheffield or London, they emerged as the popular focus for resistance to the new-right enterprise. In the case of the Greater London Council, led by the outspoken Ken Livingstone, or 'Red Ken' as he was frequently portrayed by the tabloids, the government simply ordered its abolition, leaving the capital city without an overall elected administration. Once it was established that such draconian action could be taken with minimal political fall-out, the process was repeated to abolish all the large metropolitan councils which were also under Labour control. And everywhere, local authorities were successively stripped of their powers and subjected to increasing central financial and legislative control.

It was a major onslaught by the centre against the localities. Legislation entitling local-authority tenants to buy, and requiring local authorities to sell, at discounts of up to 60 per cent, local-authority housing formed the thin end of a wedge that would see the role of the local authority as housing provider dramatically reduced, to be replaced by Housing Associations under the semi-autonomous Housing Corporation as the main provider of new rented housing for the poor. In education, under the rhetoric of greater 'choice', the 1988 Education Reform Act ended local authorities' powers to allocate places in schools, required them to devolve budgets to individual school governing bodies, and allowed schools to 'opt out' of local-authority control altogether, with their finances instead provided directly from central government. The introduction of a national curriculum with its compulsory programmes of study, and of a national system of tests equally ruled out local variation. The following year polytechnic education was taken out of local-authority control, followed by further education and sixth-form colleges in 1993. It was however through the imposition of new regulations on local-authority finance that some of the greatest centralisation was to take place. Forbidden by law, for example, to spend the receipts from their forced sale of council housing, local authorities' powers to raise local revenue were even further circumscribed as central government imposed a 'cap' on the spending that each council would be allowed, while increasing revenue was directed through central government itself. In 1987 the central state provided 40 per cent of local-authority expenditure, with strict limitations on its use attached; by 1995 this had risen to 80 per cent, while the remainder was capped.

One consequence of the stripping away of power and resources from locally elected bodies has been the mushrooming of quangos: non-elected bodies appointed by central government to oversee public services and functions in everything from the funding of schools and colleges to programmes for urban regeneration. In 1979 the new Thatcher government had railed against what it saw as the quango culture, promising to slash their numbers as part of its drive against the overweening power of the state. But the lure of political appointment and the desire to reduce the role of elected bodies that might conflict with central-government policy proved irresistible. There are many examples of this process. Take the transformation of police authorities under the 1994 Police and Magistrates Court Act which severed their traditional link with local government and reconstituted them as free-standing quangos. By the end of 1994 the new police authorities had not only a reduced involvement of local elected councillors, who had previously comprised two-thirds of the membership, but included in their 194 appointments over eighty representatives of business. According to David Shattock, then Chief Constable of Avon and Somerset, the changes meant that 'the concept of local direction and control is to a larger degree fictional' (*Statewatch*, March/April 1995: 10). In the particular case of the Metropolitan Police (which had previously been accountable directly to the Home Secretary) an advisory Police Committee was created:

> In December [1994] Mr. Howard, the Home Secretary, appointed Sir John Quinton to chair the Committee. The appointment was immediately criticised by London local councillors. Sir John does not live in London but in Buckinghamshire and has no experience of policing matters although he has extensive knowledge of the setting of budgets and monitoring performance. He is a former

chairman of Barclays Bank and a non-executive chairman of
Wimpey, the building giant.

(ibid.)

Such examples abound in the re-tooling of the British state over the
past two decades. It is not just an onslaught on hard-fought-for local
democracy, but in the endless appointment of representatives of the
business community there is an implicit privileging of business expertise
and knowledge over all other forms of understanding, especially those
which are rooted in public service. Ryan (1998) provides a useful illus-
trative case study of this process with respect to changes in British
higher education during the 1980s and 1990s, when successive
Conservative governments insisted that universities should be structured and operate as businesses. In the course of his analysis, Ryan
draws out a highly significant and common theme to the Thatcherite
transformation of the state which involved sweeping away (if possible)
all forms of opposition, whether real or imagined. In the case of British
universities, their problem was precisely that they did not look like businesses and were held to be intrinsically anti-enterprise or at least
questioning with respect to the privileging of business knowledge:

> The rhetoric of national needs and societal impatience so exem-
> plarily deployed by Mr. Waldegrave [the Conservative government
> minister then responsible for higher education] turned out to be
> covering an aggressive political strategy derived from the
> Thatcherite analysis of the obstacles to governability. Mrs
> Thatcher's government sought to destroy the 'privileges' of estab-
> lished institutions so as to enlarge the relative weight of the
> governing party . . . [It] meant that the government could shackle
> these recalcitrantly expensive institutions with ways of working
> which would both drive up the indicators of university 'productiv-
> ity' and also symbolically reinforce the work ethic of the Factory
> System. This in turn would reinforce their claim to be the guardians
> of what they declared was the true economic interest of the
> nation – the culture of enterprise – and thus secure their re-election
> as the only party fit to govern.

(Ryan 1998: 30)

Over the past two decades the face of public administration in Britain
has been transformed. The notion of public service has been replaced
with the profit-and-loss accountancy of the market. The accountability
of public officials to the public they purportedly serve has disappeared

in a morass of largely secretive appointments, in which the self-pro-claimed 'great and the good' mutually reinforce each other's power and control over large areas of public life. The influence of ordinary citizens, as elected councillors, representatives of workforces and trade unions, or consumers and recipients of services, has been drastically curtailed. If the intent of the neo-liberal project was to depoliticise public life – to remove state activity and decisions from the glare of political debate and conflict – it has secured a remarkable advance.

By 1996 the number of non-elected bodies with members appointed by central government had increased from 2,000 to 7,700, responsible for £54 billion or nearly a quarter of all public expenditure. Political appointees now outnumber elected local councillors by two to one. As Simon Jenkins has argued:

> To say that they are more accountable is absurd . . . They are mostly proxies for central government control . . . . Britain has a more cen-tralised public administration than anywhere else in the western world. In 1900 the people of London elected 12,000 people to run their city. Roughly the same number run London today, but only 2,000 are elected, while 10,000 are appointed by Downing Street.
>
> (*Telegraph* 1 February 1995)

Throughout other western democracies the number of elected officials per voter ranges from at best 1:250, to at worst 1:450; Britain, arguably the most centralised state in the western world, stands out also as the least democratic, with a ratio of 1:2,200 (ibid.).

## Taming the 'new class'

While the structure and administration of the state was subject to the anti-democratic and authoritarian discipline of the new right, the prac-tice of the welfare professionals whom the new right had identified both as a major target of and as a potential obstacle to the transfor-mation of the welfare state presented further problems. Constituted as a sizeable bloc of informed and more or less educated opinion, the pro-fessional middle classes, if not the anti-capitalist and revolutionary vanguard that they were sometimes portrayed as being, at least demanded rational discussion and debate informed by a body of knowl-edge as a basis for their actions. Largely schooled within the institutions and ethos of the welfare state itself, their influence was seen as dispro-portionate to their numbers: as teachers in schools, colleges and universities, youth leaders, social workers or probation officers, they were seen as particularly influential, especially on the young. Moreover, as professionals, their activities were particularly difficult to control. Whereas it was entirely possible to impose new disciplines and managerial control on the civil service or the large state bureaucracies, welfare professionals enjoyed a high degree of autonomy in core aspects of their work. What went on between teachers and pupils in the classroom, or social workers and clients in confidential interviews, was not something that could easily be regulated by line managers or made subject to direct state control. While this self-regulation of professionals had operated largely successfully within the welfare state without challenging its limited parameters, the new-right agenda was to call for their further curtailment and subordination to government policy (Jones and Novak 1993).

During the 1980s the welfare professions were subject to a sustained barrage of criticism, ridicule and abuse. Most of this took place through the pages of the tabloid newspapers, but not infrequently it saw government ministers lend their weight to the onslaught. Teachers for example were regularly lambasted as inefficient and ineffectual, preoccupied in the words of the Prime Minister herself with 'fashionable theories and progressive clap-trap' (cited Levitas 1986: 7) that undermined educational attainment and encouraged a disrespect for authority, and obsessed with a 'political correctness' that supposedly scorned family values and 'the British way of life' while encouraging homosexuality, sexual permissiveness and multiculturalism. Social workers similarly were regularly held up to scorn, caricatured in the *Daily Mail* as 'abusers of authority, hysterical and malignant callow youngsters who absorb moral-free marxoid and sociological theories' to undermine the family and encourage welfare dependency (cited Franklin 1989: 2).

There are various interconnected strands to these attacks on state welfare professionals and occupations. At one level it was a straightforward process of scapegoating, with state employees taking the rap for problems and failures which were far more complex than the charge of professional incompetence laid at their door. But the criticisms raised against teachers or social workers often also revealed an underlying conflict of politics, understanding and approach that was to see the welfare professions demonised in pursuit of the neo-liberal agenda.

This conflict was epitomised in the Cleveland scandal of 1988 when social workers and medical professionals took over 100 children into the temporary care of the state on the suspicion that they had been sexually abused within their families. Although most of the suspicions were later confirmed, the professionals concerned were immediately subjected to a sustained and vicious assault in the tabloid press, supported by government ministers, depicting them as witches who had deliberately set out to discredit and undermine the institution of the family in pursuit of feminist 'political correctness'. Thus the *Sunday Express* warned of 'the prevalence of ultra-feminists and of anti-family views in some medical and social work circles . . . Persons holding such views are quite unsuited to be social workers' (cited Franklin 1989: 8). As Campbell (1988) revealed in her account of Cleveland, this vilification of welfare professionals had as much to do with their challenge to wider policy imperatives as with their actual practice in Cleveland. For the Cleveland case emerged at precisely the time when government ministers were arguing that the weakness of the family institution was in large measure due to the absence of fathers. Without fathers, children were deemed to lack discipline and control and hence were more likely to become delinquent and anti-social members of an 'underclass'. At the same moment that the government and its supporters were reifying fathers and fatherhood, here was a group of state professionals pointing out in a most graphic manner that fathers even in the most 'normal' of families can also be a major problem and threat to families and their children. Hence the campaign of insults and the professional discrediting of the key participants who were recast as the problem:

> Social workers found themselves politically as well as professionally besieged. Child sex abuse was, quite correctly, perceived by people opposed to the diagnosis as no longer belonging to a populist politics of hanging and flogging but to a politics with a critique of patriarchy and power in the family.
>
> (Campbell 1988: 139)

Such attacks were part and parcel of the more general denigration of the welfare state and contributed to the notion that nothing of value could be expected from those who worked within it. This theme was similarly evident in the range of 'charters' which were introduced under the governments of John Major in the early 1990s. The implicit message of these initiatives was that welfare professionals were not to be trusted. This is part of a process of delegitimisation and silencing which is often most focused on those such as social workers, probation officers and teachers who through their work are sometimes well placed to remark upon the consequences of enduring poverty and growing inequalities.

It is difficult to assess the full impact of this ideological onslaught on the practice of welfare professionals: many were thrown onto the defensive, sometimes having difficulty to justify their work in the face of simplistic nostrums that what young offenders needed was a 'short, sharp shock' or that schools should simply instruct children what is right and wrong. Many also became increasingly demoralised at the lack of support and the constant undermining of their position. The immediate consequence in areas such as social work, however, was the adoption of tighter procedures that often worked against the interests and wishes of clients. In the face of sustained criticism of social work in the media and in parliament the response of many employing authorities was to institute procedures and practices designed to protect themselves from further criticism and attack. In the place of calculated risks and judgement – an essential feature of the work social workers are called upon to do – employers demanded the following of set procedures. One experienced social worker in a children and families team reported that due to the pressure of media attention 'and the endless re-examination of practice . . . the response from within the system has been to take out a Place of Safety Order, just in case, in order to cover your back. At least this is the advice of management' (cited NALGO 1989: 50). Another local-authority social worker in the North of England described her experience like this:

> The Department works at covering its back, and the workers work at covering their backs, and that's constantly what you are doing: to make sure that 'Yes, the child is safe'. But what's always in the back of your mind is that you might be the next poor sod who's on the front of the *Daily Mirror*.
>
> (Novak and Sennett 1996: 77)

This defensive practice – the constant covering of people's backs – is not informed by the needs of clients but by the need to protect social-services departments from criticism, and increasingly to protect the budget in what has become a resources-led provision. Another child-care worker complained that the shift in her work towards an emphasis on 'decisiveness', with fostering and adoption preferred to an attempt at rehabilitation of children with their birth families, was dictated by agency requirements rather than her clients' needs:

> Adoption is not only cheaper, it is also cleaner for the social worker – and a 'happy ending', a completed piece of work. Prevention on the other hand, is never ending, often stressful, and with current resources a continuous struggle where results are difficult to prove.
>
> (ibid.)

These kinds of development have contributed to the deteriorating relationship between state social workers and their clients. But changes in welfare practice have not only been the result of public and media criticism. In important ways changing what welfare professionals thought proved less important as a means of control than changing what they did. In true materialist fashion, government from the mid-1980s onwards embarked upon a wholesale reorganisation of professional practice and training that would transform the nature of state welfare activity and lead to a routing of the welfare professions as a potential countervailing force.

## A permanent revolution

During the past fifteen years professional welfare practice with the poor has been transformed. Scarcely a year has passed without new legislation redefining the roles and responsibilities of social workers or introducing new structures, content and processes in the education system. Just as the civil service has been subject to new managerial controls, so too previously autonomous welfare professionals have been subjected to the imposition of managerial authority. The structures and organisation of the institutions in which they work have been endlessly reorganised, and professional training has been subjected to centralised control, stripped of its potential for critical questioning and subjected to the requirements of their managerial employers. This has amounted to a permanent revolution in professional welfare activity that has disarmed opposition as workers have struggled to keep pace with the barrage of change, and that has reduced professional judgement and freedom to the proletarianised carrying-out of state policy. As the practice of those such as social workers has been changed, so the clients with whom they work have come to experience a system that is less responsive, more regulating and antagonistic.

The pace of change imposed across the welfare state was staggering and left many of those working in the system both bewildered and exhausted. Some sense of this was provided by the headteacher of a junior school in Yorkshire:

> It's so overloaded. Then they suggest teachers are failing in their job, when what they've set us is far too huge a task. It's caused stress for teachers, and it's raised this perception in parents that schools aren't coping – when they introduced a system that could never be coped with in the first place. But I think it's like the miners' strike. I think it's sinister. I think it was planned this way, to

swamp the system, and after that they can do what they want – which is to undermine local government and take control of the funding and the curriculum. Then they're dictating all the moves aren't they ?

(cited Davies 1998: 77)

Another headteacher similarly described his school as now 'buried in bumf' which he says 'just keeps coming by every post':

Conscious he is living through a moment of history, the headmaster has begun taking his own photographs. He arranged his weekly post on two tables and recorded this for his governors; when the papers for the new tests for seven year olds came, he had a child pose beside them and the parcel was a third of her size.

(*Guardian* 8 February 1992)

The teaching profession was one of the early targets for reform. Berated as obsessed with trendy fashions and opinion dating from the 1960s, and with teaching methods 'in which', according to Margaret Thatcher, 'the old virtues of discipline and self-restraint were denigrated' (cited Levitas 1986: 7), methods of child-centred education were criticised amongst claims of falling standards and demands for a return to traditional forms of whole-class rather than individual child-centred teaching. Exploration and questioning were to be replaced with rote learning and certainty through methods based on discipline and control. The introduction of a National Curriculum for schools in the 1988 Education Reform Act was to codify a new educational content that teachers would be required to follow. State schools (although significantly not the private schools favoured by the wealthy) would now, and for the first time, be required to follow a centrally prescribed syllabus. Backed up by a new national inspectorate, and the compulsory testing of all children at the ages of 7, 11, 14 and 16 in the core subjects that the National Curriculum prescribed, teacher autonomy was significantly curtailed.

Central to the taming of the welfare professions, as in every sphere of state employment, has been the imposition of new forms of managerial control (Clarke and Newman 1997). This has involved not only bringing into the public services managers from the private sector, but also and crucially an assertion of managers' 'right to manage' against the contrary advice of those who carry out the work. 'It's management from the top down,' argued one social worker, 'we are simply instructed to do things: "This is as it is, this is the reality, so don't bother arguing on behalf of your clients; don't bother objecting on professional grounds, because this is what you're expected to do"' (cited Novak and Sennett 1996: 73). What previously existed as a stratum within welfare agencies of professional supervision and support for front-line workers has thus been realigned as a process of management supervision and control. 'There's less emphasis now on support and help', said one social worker, 'and more about surveying what you do' (ibid.).

From the point of view of managers what has become the over-riding objective is not the delivery of a responsive and appropriate service, but the need to work within a budget. In the view of another social worker, 'there's like an inquisition in management: a sort of semi-punitive "there is only this much; you will continue to make savings; you will cut back; you will insist on cheaper alternatives, or you will just refuse applications for money"' (cited Novak and Sennett 1996: 72). Significantly, the devolution of budgets lower down the hierarchy that has accompanied this process, justified in terms of greater responsiveness and 'choice', has had the effect of implicating professionals themselves in rationing resources. Those who previously would have argued on behalf of their clients now find their professional judgements constrained by the need to balance the accounts. Another social worker put this in familiar terms: 'you might as well do it yourself rather than have someone else do it. Do you want to have it done to you, or do you want to have some say over how it's done? I think that's the only way I can rationalise it' (cited Novak and Sennett 1996: 73). According to Bob Holman:

> New Right managerialism entails centralised organisations where profit-oriented managers set targets for lower staff to meet within set budgets. Translated into social work the results are highly paid directors, often with no recent experience of grass-roots practice, devising procedures for those at the hard end. Such an approach and ethos have little in common with community social work, which stresses user involvement in decision making and which campaigns against the very inequalities which affluent directors now reinforce.
>
> (*Guardian* 20 January 1993)

Alongside the introduction of a new managerialism has also come a vastly increased body of inspection and audit. This combination of managerialism and audit – whether in the form of OFSTED inspections of schools or the internal inspection and quality assurance units which have mushroomed throughout the public sector – has in little over a decade brought about unprecedented change in the control of state workers which has been crucial to the re-tooling of the state. According to Ryan:

> As with Henry VIII, the new power needed a new kind of law, and thus new magistrates. The New Public Management is the new magistracy: audit is their law. The functionality of audit to the new political class is that it constructs political power while appearing to secure the ends of justice and economy. As Michael Power has so lucidly shown, an audit system constructs auditability, by that very fact curtailing the discretions and privileges long enjoyed by professionals, even when employed by the state. Audit reconstructs institutions, away from collegiality towards line management and upward accountability . . . It is the ultimate divide-and-rule technique for the age of measurement. As with Solon and Henry VIII, only the law givers are not subject to audit.
>
> (Ryan 1998: 32)

At the same time legislation has been introduced redefining what social workers are required and expected to do. The 1990 National Health Service and Community Care Act was one of the most significant, as a result of which social workers were no longer to have a major role as providers of care, but instead have come to act as purchasers of care from the private sector. In this their relationships with clients have also changed: the task of social-work intervention is now increasingly to assess clients' needs, not help them to solve their problems. When the results of these assessments have to be translated into 'packages of care' purchased from an over-stretched budget, the potential for distrust and conflict is significantly increased. The introduction of the Children Act provides another example of the way in which the increased proceduralisation of professional practice contributes to an atmosphere of antagonism. In the view of one child-care worker:

> The changes that have been most obvious have been in the legal and court arena . . . it's more visible, more high profile, more testing of your every move . . . They're asking for expert opinions to test our opinions; if they're getting an expert, we'll get an expert, and the parents' solicitors get an expert in: you might get three experts, so then you're rummaging around the country looking for experts . . . It's much more confrontational, much more adversarial and much more legally driven.
>
> (cited Novak and Sennett 1996: 76)

The detailed report prepared by the Children's Rights Development Unit (1994) on the position of children in Britain likewise noted that the preventive work promised by the 1989 Children Act was in most areas of the country non-existent and that in the face of budgetary constraints priority was given to the surveillance of families where there was a suspicion of child abuse. What was absent, they argued, was any significant support to parents. As the *Guardian* noted in reviewing research in this area, 'child protection workers are spending most of their time policing the parenting habits of extremely disadvantaged people who need practical support more than surveillance' (*Guardian* 30 March 1994).

As Bill Jordan has noted, the already strained relationships which existed between clients and social-work agencies have thus been stretched even further:

> This is particularly clear in the field of child care . . . Obviously, as clients' plights have become more desperate, and as they identify social workers more with the state agencies which do not meet their needs, the chances of co-operation are reduced; but the evidence points also to more punitive ideologies among social workers, more social distance between them and their clientele, and a greater emphasis on decisiveness, which often works against partnership and sharing.
>
> (Jordan 1988: 345)

That some social workers might, as a number did, question and challenge these developments was further to put the spotlight on the existing systems of professional training and education. In the words of the then Chief Inspector of the Social Services Inspectorate, Sir William Utting, 'there is an unacceptable degree of pretentiousness in social work that can be dangerous. The professionally qualified social worker is in as much need of regulation as the unqualified worker' (cited Fry 1991: 21).

During the early 1990s, following substantial changes to the system of teacher training, social-work training was also to be subject to the now familiar process of public criticism and reform. Much of the criticism centred on what was seen as the inappropriate and disproportionate amount of social-science teaching in the social-work curriculum: a factor that was seen as encouraging newly qualified professionals to question public policy and its consequences for the poor. Timothy Yeo, for example – a junior Conservative minister in 1992 – complained that social-work education was far too preoccupied with 'ologies and isms'

(*Independent* 13 December 1992). In the same vein Virginia Bottomley, then Secretary of State for Health, announced in a speech to the Conservative Local Government conference in February 1994 that there 'will be no place for trendy theories' or 'the theory that "isms" or "ologies" come before common sense and practical skills' (Bottomley 1994). These 'practical skills' are now embodied in the form of 'competencies' that form the basis of the new reduced professional training for social workers. Derived from an analysis of what social workers are expected to do by their employing authorities (who now take equal place alongside educators in the management and design of professional training courses), they are explicitly task-oriented, while social science has been relegated to the margins.

The cumulative effect of these changes has been significantly to reduce the professional autonomy of those who work within the welfare services. For many this has led to disillusionment and a sense that they have little to offer: a feeling common among workers and clients alike. Some sense of this is provided by Oppenheim in his account of social work in a particularly impoverished part of London:

> Gatekeeping is no longer subtle; we lock the front doors and if needs be put on the answerphone. The effect is frustrating for consumers and workers; anger is seemingly more in evidence and so is desperation . . . There are many children in care without allocated workers: without, let me stress, allocated parents. I now often consider an admission to care more an abuse than remaining at home. . . . Supervision orders are left to languish, as are the kids at the back of them. Social enquiry reports often cannot be completed in Haringey, due to severe staff cuts and local union action over unallocated work. The result for kids and their families; no result . . . The freezing of aids and adaptations budgets means that clients already waiting 18 months for an occupational therapy service cannot have one after all. The effect then is a state of depression and demoralisation amongst staff everywhere; people are desperate to leave and go to another authority.
>
> (Oppenheim 1987: 10–11)

For those who remain, professional practice is no longer what it was: 'I'm not sure what we've turned into,' is the bleak view of one social worker, 'I'm not sure where it's taking us – or what we're becoming. I don't think it was what was had in mind at the end of the war with the Beveridge Report. It's a welfare state that has changed beyond recognition' (cited Novak and Sennett 1996: 78). Yet, for all the change, social work remains, and it is in this that the transformation of the state needs to be understood. It is not simply that the welfare state has been dismantled: significant parts of it may have disappeared, but others have been turned into something else. According to one social worker, 'I think the role of social services has even more become a policing one in terms of policing the poor . . . It is a very easy thing to do, far easier than most members of the public know' (ibid.). Another summed up the situation more precisely:

> We have seen fifteen years or whatever of a government trying to revert back to less government intervention; yet there are certain mechanisms of the state that are intervening far more than ever before – and I'd say that we were one of them.
>
> (ibid.)

## The abandonment of reason

Behind many of the developments discussed above lay a profound anti-intellectualism that increasingly came to influence policy-making and that continues to have profound and disturbing implications for its future. Policy and practice were no longer to be informed by accumulated knowledge and research but by the creation of a new 'common sense' based on a narrow morality and 'traditional values'. It was this that formed the basis for John Major's ill-fated 'back to basics' initiative in the early 1990s, derailed by a series of sexual scandals amongst members of his own cabinet. But the real significance of the 'back to basics' message was not that of personal sexual behaviour. According to the Downing Street Policy Unit briefing paper which preceded its announcement, there was a need to frame policies according to 'traditional values [and] common sense', and this required a challenge to 'a number of the social orthodoxies that took root in the 1960s', particularly in 'those areas of social policy where theorists dragged professionals and administrators furthest from common sense' (*Guardian* 6 November 1993).

The easy and often simplistic 'common-sense' explanations of social issues and problems were thus to be pitched against theory and the role of intellectuals in the analysis and framing of policy. Frequently this has involved a belittling of those who do not support the new orthodoxy. As Melanie Phillips, for example, argued:

> There is a conspiracy of silence about the underclass . . . British

social scientists, who are liberally-minded almost to a man or woman, recoil so sharply from the stigma and blame attached to Murray's analysis that you feel they'd rather burn their gowns and mortar boards before admitting that something similar might be happening here too.

(BBC Radio 4 Analysis 3 December 1992)

Used as a way to sideline alternative explanations and prescriptions, it has also been used to elevate 'practical experience' over knowledge and research. 'We don't believe Whitehall knows best,' argued Tony Blair, 'we need practical experience. We need the insights of people who have worked at the sharp end' (Blair 1997b). While those working at the sharp end may indeed have insights to contribute, the development of policy based on existing practice also stifles alternative approaches. The straitjacket imposed on professional education and training by the demand that it now be relevant only to the task in hand, as we have seen, leaves the purpose of that task unquestioned.

In the face of contrary explanations or in order to avoid entanglement with often complex debates, leading politicians have argued that their prescriptions for action were not clouded by the views of so-called experts but rooted in simple, self-evident truths: 'You can argue forever about the causes of crime. My approach is based on some simple moral principles. That children – at home and at school – must be taught the difference between right and wrong' (Michael Howard, October 1993, cited Goldson 1999: 10). In similar fashion, John Patten, then a junior Home Office minister, declared,

> I have got more impatient with the analysis of why people commit crime. Five years ago we were told it was the Tories in power and it was unemployment, now the Tories are in power and it's affluence that causes crime. All these things are absurd. In the end people commit crime because they are bad.
>
> (cited May 1991: 109)

In the face of such simplistic principles, the advocates of the disciplinary state certainly do not want to be reminded by the likes of social workers that families are paradoxical institutions – places of love as well as abuse – or that most families and households are not defeated by moral relativism but by unrelenting social and economic difficulties which make their tasks increasingly impossible (Seabrook 1998: 38–9). Theories, and especially those informed by a critical understanding of the social world, are dangerous and unsettling to the new moral certainties.

If theory was no longer to inform policy, then neither was research, or at least neither was research that challenged government perceptions and dogma. The denigration of intellectual enquiry in general and of social science in particular as the special pleading of the 'new class' and as irrelevant to a social policy driven by moral imperatives was to see countless reports on social and economic conditions dismissed, side-lined and ridiculed. Even statistical information produced by the government itself, which might have provided ammunition for its opponents or even acted as the basis for a rational review of state policy, failed to escape untouched. As early as 1981 the 'efficiency' review of civil-service operations conducted on behalf of the government by Derek Rayner had recommended a 40 per cent cut in the budget and staffing of the social-survey division of the Office of Population Censuses and Surveys. According to the *Times*, this would

> cut the provision of politically sensitive figures like the size of the NHS waiting list and private patients' use of NHS facilities, and reduce information available to MPs, select committees, royal commissions and the Public Accounts Committee . . . Annual social security statistics would not be published unless sales covered costs.
>
> (*Times* 11 March 1981)

A month later the government published a White Paper outlining the changes to be made:

> Changes to the Government's statistical service would include stopping all work on wealth distribution and reducing the frequency of income distribution. There would be less frequent collection of housing and employment statistics and substantial changes in data collected on health.
>
> (*Times* 30 April 1981)

By 1997 there had been thirty-two changes in the basis for the calculation of unemployment statistics: a sleight of hand that not only reduced significantly the numbers that would count as unemployed, but would even render official statistics useless for official purposes. As the Department of Education and Employment was forced to admit in an application to the European Commission for funding based on the numbers unemployed, 'while a useful indicator of labour market trends, the claimant count is not adequate for the purpose' (*Observer* 20 April 1997). According to Melanie Phillips:

The continuing abuse of national statistics is a prime example of the way market forces have helped destroy the ethos of public service. 'Value for money' is a euphemism for stifling information which properly belongs to the public . . . The threat is merely a symptom of a much wider and deeper malaise. In the mid-eighties the statistical service fell victim to two Thatcherite mind-sets. The first was the obsession with cutting costs, the result of which was that statistics became unreliable as standards took a dive. The second was even more destructive: the identification of the Conservative Party with the state, and the resulting erosion throughout Whitehall of the concept of a public interest standing aloof from party politics. The effect of this was that Ministers now wanted neither objective policy advice from civil servants nor objective facts from researchers.

(*Observer* 23 March 1997)

During the 1990s this repudiation of alternative knowledge and research became most apparent, although not exclusively, in the development of penal policy and in the assertion of the Home Secretary, despite the available evidence, that 'prison works'. Thus in 1994, following media suggestions that a hard core of 'persistent offenders' were responsible for the majority of juvenile crime, the government passed new legislation allowing for the incarceration of 12- to 15-year-old 'persistent offenders' in secure training units, and announced an increase in the number of places from 295 to 665, despite research funded by the Home Office which showed that such offenders were responsible for at most 10 per cent of juvenile crime, and that the crimes they committed were no more serious than average (*Guardian* 18 February 1994). Other reports contrary to the drift of government policy were simply shelved or never published. In 1995 the *Guardian* reported on a series of Home Office research studies with the potential to undermine government pronouncements and policies in areas as diverse as the inability of courts to deal with bail bandits, the assumed economic motivation of asylum seekers and the criminal propensity of black youths, all of which had been shelved without publication. According to Harry Fletcher of the National Association of Probation Officers, 'most of these reports have been completed for a year or more. Some have a crucial bearing on policy. The real reason for delay is political expediency' (*Guardian* 26 February 1995). Following a fact-finding mission to the United States in May 1994 by three senior civil servants, which questioned the proposed introduction in Britain of US-style 'boot camps' as expensive and ineffective failures, the Home

Office refused to release their report to Parliament on the grounds that it was confidential advice to ministers (*Independent* 14 March 1995).

Where the government was unable to prevent the flow of evidence that demonstrated that Britain was becoming a more divided society or that the authoritarian drift of state welfare was destroying the well-being of increasing numbers of people, it resorted increasingly to derision. Whether it was the Archbishop of Canterbury's Commission report *Faith in the City* (1985) or the Rowntree Foundation's enquiry into income and wealth, ministers and their tabloid supporters degraded the issues and debates, challenged the credentials of those who had produced the reports, and questioned their motives for doing so. Calls for an end to the reification of the market as the key driver of social development and demands for a legitimate and positive role for the state in the mediation of market forces and the protection of the most vulnerable were casually and consistently dismissed. Those who questioned or challenged government policy were commonly presented as dinosaurs who had failed to come to terms with the new realities. When, for example, a United Nations panel reviewed Britain's perfor-mance in complying with the UN Convention on Children's Rights – which Margaret Thatcher had signed in a blaze of publicity in April 1990 – and revealed that the plight of many children in Britain had sig-nificantly worsened as a consequence of policies implemented since 1979, the government reacted with utter outrage and newspapers dis-missed the review with typical xenophobia. As the leader writer of the *Daily Mail* argued, the UN Committee's work was a 'waste of money and . . . sheer impudence when members coming from places such as Egypt and the Philippines see fit to rebuke the UK Government for fail-ing in its responsibilities to guarantee children's rights' (*Daily Mail* 28 January 1995).Yet as the Children's Rights Development Unit (1994: 71) noted, the evidence for the UN's conclusions was compelling, revealing as it did that no country had experienced such a huge increase in inequality as had Britain between 1979 and 1995, with more than 4 million children living in homes below the European poverty line (half the national average income).

## Towards a penal state

In 1993 David Faulkner, Deputy Secretary at the Home Office and the civil servant in charge of criminal justice policy between 1982 and 1990, wrote an article in the *Guardian* in which he reflected on his recent experience:

The government's change of direction in its policies on crime and criminal justice is probably the most sudden and the most radical which has ever taken place in this area of public policy. Until a year ago, these policies had evolved gradually, largely driven by consultation with professionals, practitioners, academics and representatives of informed opinion . . . Within a period of less than twelve months, much of the programme has been politically discredited and seems to have been largely abandoned.

(*Guardian* 11 November 1993)

Arguing that 'there is now a serious void at the centre of the criminal justice system', he noted how this was being filled by increasingly authoritarian measures and policies:

Overwhelming emphasis is now being placed on criminalisation, detection, conviction and punishment as the means of dealing not only with violence and other forms of serious crime, but also with what has previously been regarded (not always universally) as anti-social behaviour, for example squatting or interference with fox hunting.

(ibid.)

What has characterised this authoritarian drift is the view that criminalisation and imprisonment is an effective and appropriate response to a wide range of social conflicts and problems. Encapsulated in the Conservative Home Secretary Michael Howard's oft-repeated slogan that 'prison works' it is a policy that has been pursued in defiance of evidence, even from the Home Office itself, to the contrary. Two years after Michael Howard announced his new tough approach to crime at the 1993 Conservative Party conference, the prison population stood at its highest ever recorded level of 51,000; by the late 1990s it was over 64,000, and officially projected to rise to 92,000 by the year 2005. On a seemingly relentless trajectory of growth, Britain now has one of the highest rates of imprisonment in the developed world, dwarfed in numbers only by the USA.

As with the USA, these trends stand in contrast to the experience of other developed societies. As Allan Levy QC noted, compared to other countries in western Europe, Britain is notable, for example, in lowering the age of criminal responsibility as the trend elsewhere has been in the opposite direction. 'It seems extraordinary', he wrote, 'that while many other countries advance both their thinking and the age of criminal responsibility, we spend a generation failing to do either' (*Guardian* 24

November 1994). In Britain plans for new children's prisons are proceeding despite the change of government. These prisons are intended to hold up to forty children aged between 12 and 14 years of age who have committed three or more offences. They are deliberately intended to be tough places:

> The draft rules for these institutions have been powerfully criticised by Frances Crook, director of the Howard League for Penal Reform. She noted that the original draft referred to 'children'. This was apparently unacceptable to ministers and was altered to 'trainees'. The rules as to punishment, restraint, visiting, family contact and communications with the outside world are unacceptable by the standards of the Children Act regulations for residential care and the European Convention on Human Rights. No lessons have been learnt from recent scandals, including Pindown.
>
> (Allan Levy, *Guardian* 24 November 1994)

In the face of the seemingly inexorable rise in imprisonment, even the Director General of the Prison Service, Richard Tilt, felt compelled in 1997 to sound a note of alarm. 'People ought to question whether this is the best way to spend public money,' he said, 'some of the people coming into prison could be dealt with as effectively in the community and at a very much lower cost. I am worried about the size of the prison population and the rate at which it is expanding' (cited *Economist* 15 March 1997). Similarly the Secretary General of the Prison Governors' Association, arguing that 'a number of women in prison are there as a direct result of poverty and abuse', went on to point out:

> Prison governors have been aware for some years that imprisonment is being over-used. This impacts particularly on women, because the growth of the female prison population has been double that of the male population over the past three years, and there has been no corresponding increase in the number of offences being committed by women.
>
> (*Guardian* 25 March 1998)

The rapid expansion of imprisonment symbolises the growing authoritarianism of state policy, targeted overwhelmingly at the most vulnerable and impoverished. But it is also symptomatic of a wider trend that has seen the criminal law brought to bear on an increasing range of social issues, and of the use of policing to combat the consequences of a divided society. The police themselves are divided over these developments, thrust as they are into a more overtly antagonistic relationship with wider groups of the population. As one police constable with twenty-two years' service saw it, 'morale has been going down gradually for a while . . . I think it's because we don't know what we are supposed to be doing any more. We are being asked to sort out problems that should be done by other people – the council, the social services' (*Independent* 1 December 1991). John Alderson, the former Chief Constable of Devon and Cornwall and a long-standing liberal voice within police circles, has also recognised that the criminal justice system is being used to manage the social problems of a polarised society and expressed considerable alarm on the grounds that this is leading to a considerable diminution in civil liberties:

> The [then] Home Secretary Michael Howard deals with social problems in a simplistic way by passing a law making an activity illegal and then asking for policemen to enforce that law. 'Give me your liberties and I will protect you' is the language of dictators.
>
> (Alderson 1996: 11)

Being a former chief constable makes Alderson's comments especially significant. He is one of the few senior police officers to have expressed concern about the authoritarian drift in the state apparatus and he has been especially alarmed by the extended role given to the secret service, MI5, in domestic policing:

> It is fatal to let the secret service into the area of ordinary crime. MI5 are not under the same restraints as the police. They infiltrate organisations, people's jobs and lives. They operate almost like a cancer, infiltrating and destroying trust and security between people. Howard is putting the building blocks in place for an East German style Stasi-like force where half the population finishes up spying on the other half.
>
> (Alderson 1996: 11–12)

That the powers of the secret state are extensive and widely used is not in doubt. Nor is the fact that members of the police and security services frequently, and routinely, exceed the powers allowed to them by law. Periodically the use of these extra-legal powers is regularised. Thus the 1996 Police Act gave police the legal power to enter anyone's home or workplace and to hide surveillance devices on the permission of a chief constable (rather than, as previously allowed, only under the authorisation of the courts) where there was suspicion of 'serious crime' (a definition which includes any crime which 'involves the use of violence, results in substantial financial gain, or is conducted by a large number of persons in pursuit of a common purpose'). This was one of a number of pieces of legislation which New Labour in opposition declined to oppose; indeed Jack Straw welcomed it as putting established police practice on a legal basis. 'The police have been doing this for years,' he said, 'now they will be supervised. They will be more accountable' (*Independent* 5 January 1997).

As these powers have been extended, so they have come increasingly to mesh with the extended powers of a centralised state in areas such as immigration control or the investigation of benefit fraud. The 1997 Social Security Administration (Fraud) Act, for example, extends the powers of the Department of Social Security to obtain any information held by the Inland Revenue or Customs and Excise, or to obtain information held by people working for other government departments which relates to 'passports, immigration and emigration, nationality or prisoners . . . for use in the prevention, detection, investigation or prosecution of offences relating to social security; or for use in checking the accuracy of information' (Cracknell, Jarvis and Wilson 1996: 20) and also to pass this information to local authorities in respect of the benefits they administer. It further gave power to a national inspectorate to monitor anti-fraud work by local authorities, and to allow local authorities 'to appoint inspectors from among their employees or . . . from among employees of a contractor acting on its behalf' with the power 'to enter business premises to make enquiries about any person believed to be a benefit claimant or recipient' (Cracknell, Jarvis and Wilson 1996: 25).

This surveillance now includes the use of MI5 in benefit fraud detection, and random questioning of the population. According to one report:

> Fraud investigators from the Benefits Agency are interrogating people stopped by police in routine roadside checks. Benefits officers accompanied police last year as they checked up to 10,000 vehicles for road worthiness and tachograph offences. After the police had finished they handed over to benefits investigators, who asked drivers and passengers if they were claiming benefit. In one case a woman claiming benefit was stopped and asked numerous questions. When she said her children were being looked after by her sister the investigator asked for the sister's details in case she too was claiming the Jobseeker's allowance but not actively seeking work. Social Security Minister Oliver Heald commented 'Fraud

investigators identify themselves to any driver and passenger to whom they wish to speak. Drivers and passengers are informed that they are under no obligation to answer any questions, and that they are not being detained'.

(*Observer* 2 February 1997)

In the light of such developments, the drift of penal policy has been met with significant criticism from within the criminal justice system itself. The annual conference of prison governors in 1994 denounced the Home Secretary's penal policies as 'ill-considered', while according to the governor of Armley jail in Leeds, 'all we seem to get is knee-jerk reaction, expediency and dogma' (*Guardian* 10 March 1994). Judge Tumim, the Chief Inspector of Prisons, similarly described current policy as 'a depressing, backward experience' (*Telegraph* 10 March 1994). Yet it is a policy which has continued, fuelled by the Labour government's promise to be 'tough on crime'. In 1995 Jack Straw, subsequently to become Home Secretary in New Labour's 1997 government, called for measures to 'reclaim the streets for the law-abiding public citizen', identifying in particular

the obstacles faced by pedestrians and motorists in going about their daily business, the winos and addicts whose aggressive begging affronts and sometimes threatens decent compassionate citizens and the 'squeegee merchants' who wait at large road junctions to force on reticent motorists their windscreen cleaning service.

(*Independent* 5 September 1995)

Since then the use of legal sanction as a means of combating what is seen as 'anti-social' behaviour has emerged as a significant plank in New Labour policy. In his first public speech as Prime Minister, Tony Blair indicated his intention to 'enforce a new code of laws that crack down on crime and other anti-social behaviour', including proposals for the institution of curfews and greater use of the law to evict anti-social neighbours. Of particular concern was

the scourge of many communities . . . Young people with nothing to do are sucked into a life of vandalism and drugs, and make life hell for other citizens. Our Youth Offender Teams are going to nip young offending in the bud. Children wandering the streets at night, getting into trouble, growing into a life of criminality, will be subject to Child Protection Orders.

(Blair 1997b)

As even the generally right-of-centre *Economist* noted:

> Labour, intimidated by public, and tabloid newspaper, support for these policies, has not dared oppose them. But in their eagerness to outdo one another on law and order toughness, the politicians have not only ignored the expense and injustice of their prisons policy, but also overestimated its effectiveness . . . There is little proof of any simple connection between imprisonment rates and crime.
>
> (*Economist* 15 March 1997)

According to John Alderson:

> Much of the language of politicians like Howard and his Labour shadow, Jack Straw is Victorian in content. They share a moral cowardice whereby each is too scared to say anything different in case they lose votes. We should be looking for new ways of preventing crime rather than simply relying on the criminal justice system. The legal system should be the last resort if all else fails.
>
> (Alderson 1996 : 12)

There is little evidence at the time of writing that the 1997 Labour administration will attempt any significant change to the trajectory of these developments in the state. Particularly with regard to social policy and the management of inequality, Labour ministers along with their Democratic counterparts in the USA have accepted key elements of the conservative programme. In both of these societies there is a keen sense of disappointment and abandonment amongst those who looked to these political parties for a more compassionate and supportive response to the acute pressures wrought by growing inequality and poverty. For the poor and the working class more generally, the state continues to become more authoritarian and restrictive, more concerned with their control and containment and unconcerned with their worsening plight. This policing state, when compared with its immediate social-democratic predecessor, reflects an acceptance of widening social inequalities and poverty. Increasingly stripped of its positive welfare functions and abandoning any pretence of social obligation and rights, the state reverts to more draconian measures of maintaining order. The signs of this growing authoritarianism are already well established, both in Britain and in the USA. According to an editorial in the *Independent*:

> Swift justice, the death penalty, fresh powers for the FBI: Bill

Clinton's rhetoric suggests an opportunistically spotted turning point. This is the President as strong man, not abroad but at home, as paterfamilias, protector of the people. Amid the firmness, the reassuring sense of purpose, there is a hint of the authoritarian . . . Meanwhile, here in Britain, legislation eats away at civil rights. The Public Order Act is employed at Brightlingsea, where householders receive letters warning them of their limited rights to demonstrate. The Criminal Justice Act challenges the nonconformist lives of many travellers, squatters and ravers. The right to silence of suspects is curbed. Rules about disclosure of evidence are to be altered in favour of the prosecuting authorities. Ministers plan the introduction of identity cards and pursue journalists through the courts . . . On both sides of the Atlantic, governments are flexing their muscles internally, expanding their remit on law and order. As the Republicans in the US, and Labour in Britain realise, there are votes to be had in pushing the government into more draconian measures.

*(Independent* 25 April 1995)

As Nils Christie has written:

You have to ask, what are the consequences of this repressive penal policy? In some US cities it's like a war situation . . . In the US today there are one and a half million in prison and another three and a half under penal control outside prison. Nearly 5% of adult males are under penal control: it's not crime control but a kind of war situation . . . There is a war between civil society and crime control society – the state in its most primitive, punitive form.

(Christie 1996: 10–12)

# 6    Abandoning the poor

If the view of the new right was that the abandonment of the poor was good for the market, the view of New Labour would appear to be that the abandonment of the poor to the market is good for the poor. In the guise of a concern to tackle the problem of social exclusion – the term that in the New Labour vocabulary has come to replace discussion of poverty – social policies have not only continued to seek market solutions to the problems of unemployment or economic dependency; they have also been justified as in the best interests of those at whom they are directed.

It is the continuities between the policies of the new right which dominated British politics between 1979 and 1997 and of the New Labour government which replaced them that are more striking than the differences. The ideological veneer which surrounds these policies may have changed: instead of stressing the virtues of self-help and individualism, New Labour appeals to notions of community, to social responsibility, social inclusion and the need to overcome divisions. But in terms of policy and practice the trajectory remains largely the same. As Peter Mandelson, the closest political ally of New Labour's Prime Minister put it, 'New Labour's mission is to move forward from where Margaret Thatcher left off, rather than dismantle every single thing she did' (cited Gray 1998: 5).

It is not simply that the New Labour government committed itself from the start to maintaining its Conservative predecessor's restricted public-spending plans; nor that it promised not to raise taxation, and thereby begin to reverse the previous massive redistribution of resources in favour of the rich. Nor is it simply that it moved, once in office, to implement the unfinished policies of the previous Conservative government, including the imposition of cuts in benefits to lone parents and the introduction of a new, stricter regime of benefits for disabled people. It is also that its continued thinking and policies concerning the poor reveal a fundamental continuity that has dismayed and disheartened many of those who in 1997 thought that they were voting for change.

Eighteen years of one of the most dogmatic new-right governments – led for the first twelve by one of its world leaders and founder of its own creed of Thatcherism – inflicted immense damage on the economic, social, political and cultural life of Britain. The loss of manufacturing capacity, and the 2.75 million jobs that went with it, has left millions out of work, and many more who have shifted to the service industries poorer. The runaway antics of the City of London and of other global financial institutions have created what one writer called 'The Casino Economy'. Families and communities have been put under immense stress and pressure. British workers work the longest hours in Europe; many have more than one job, and most couples get by only by both of them working outside the home. To do this, if they have children, often means working different shifts in the hope that at least one will be available for childcare, and politicians and the newspapers worry about why 'family life' has deteriorated, or communities cease to hold together. People live more isolated lives, fearful of the streets, afraid of one another. The cult of the individual – 'there is no such thing as society' – has shaped for a generation its own brands of intolerance and bigotry.

Above all, the past eighteen years in Britain have witnessed the sharpest and most sustained widening of inequality of all countries in the world. Its effects on individuals and on millions is incalculable. Hunger and homelessness are now a permanent feature on British streets. Millions are over-worked, over-stressed and embattled by the struggle simply to get by. It can be counted in everything, from widening infant mortality to early death, and is the primary cause of ill health. Remarkably, millions survive with a fair degree of humour and resilience, but for others the damage to the human – and social – psyche is everywhere evident.

This calls for a programme of reconstruction: an attempt systematically and strategically to rebuild from the bottom up. But in its first year in office the new government did little, other than commit itself to following its predecessor's policies. In the meantime, the dynamics producing and widening poverty have remained.

## The third way

When President Clinton in his State of the Union message announced, 'My fellow Americans, we have found a third way' he was speaking following a series of meetings, first at Chequers and then at the White

House, between the British and US governments. These meetings, attended by senior government ministers, policy advisers and academics, were not unique, following as they did in a long tradition of both official and unofficial encounters that mark the 'special relationship' between the two countries, widely trumpeted in the affinity between Reagan and Thatcher. But they were seen as particularly important, 'underlining the growing closeness of the two, and the importance the British and US governments now place on social policy as the pre-eminent issue for centre-left governments to tackle' (Patrick Wintour, *Observer* 1 February 1998). According to the Home Secretary, Jack Straw, one of the participants, 'the two governments are learning more from one another all the time. There is now a deep ideological relationship' (cited ibid.).

This relationship has been built in part around an attempt to construct a political philosophy and agenda that defines government practice in the two countries. The third way represents the latest attempt to give this philosophy a name. Just as the new right in the 1970s felt compelled to construct a new agenda in order to distinguish itself from its predecessors, so too the third way has spawned think tanks and discussion groups in the attempt to define and flesh out this philosophy, and to create what is claimed to be the defining path for politics in the twenty-first century.

Composed of a mixture of communitarianism, the religiously inspired 'ethical socialist' traditions of the Labour Party, and a heavy emphasis on media presentation, New Labour's version of the third way seeks the advantage of a competitive capitalism without its disintegrating effects. It is, according to Peter Mandelson, 'a vision of competitiveness and social cohesion' (Mandelson 1997: 7). It is a holy grail that has eluded many in the past.

What distinguishes New Labour and its third way from the new right is principally their use of the state. For the new right state intervention was anathema: at best dispensed with altogether; at most confined to the maintenance of the infrastructure of the economy, trade, law and order and security. Faced with growing poverty and social stress, all it could do was withdraw into an increasingly coercive role. The third way allows for a more interventionist state, taking on the authoritarian legacy of its predecessors, but adding to this the greater range of powers the state possesses to achieve its ends.

These ends remain essentially the same, although they are clothed in different language and framed in different philosophies. Margaret Thatcher, for all her hankering after a return to 'Victorian values', saw her mission as to modernise British society: to shake it free of the inertia and lack of dynamism that the featherbedding of the 'nanny state' had created, and to open it to the requirements of an increasingly global capitalism. Modernisation equally remains at the heart of New Labour's project: partly in response to the failure of Thatcherism it promises a renewed determination, backed by what it sees as more appropriate policies, to achieve the same end. According to Blair, the 'next decade will be about how to recreate the bonds of civic society and community in a way compatible with the far more individualistic nature of modern, economic, social and cultural life' (Blair 1997b). It is a mission that takes a great deal for granted.

The acceptance of individualism which underpins the third way reflects Blair's earlier successes in expunging class as the basis for Labour Party mobilisation. The replacement of Clause 4 in the Labour Party's constitution was the symbolic achievement of Labour Party 'modernisation': a process that has seen it break its links with the collective organisation of workers in trade unions, and reject class (and other forms of structured) inequality both as explanation and as a basis for political practice. As in contemporary theories of postmodernism, people are identified not by their collective experiences – as workers, as women or black people – but as individuals. It is not the same individualism as that of the new right, although it draws many parallels, not least with the 'active citizens' that fleetingly formed part of John Major's agenda in the early 1990s. The new right's individualism was of the sink or swim variety. New Labour's individualism is much more actively promoted.

Without these structures, of explanation and action, the third way falls back on vague notions of community as a way to hold individuals together. 'Individuals prosper in a strong and active community of citizens', argued the Prime Minister (Blair 1997a). But communities are seen as under threat, if not actually in decline, in particular in poor communities and in the weakened hold of the family. The reconstruction of poor communities, as the cement of social order, requires the construction of new moral codes. As Anna Coote has argued:

> Communitarians, like most conservatives, maintain that society is unravelling and needs to be knitted together again. The excesses of capitalism and welfare-state liberalism have produced a wayward individualism which has loosened the bonds of family and shaken moral certainties. Society must be restored to its old self.
>
> (*Independent* 3 July 1995)

In the British context, this search for a moral order also reflects the strong strand of religious commitment evident in New Labour's leadership. It is a function of government: to establish clear (but 'modern') ideas of what is right and wrong, to construct a public morality anew, and to discipline those who err. In this New Labour draws on many now familiar themes of individual responsibility, discipline, work and the family. 'New Labour stands for the ordinary families who work hard and play by the rules', argue Mandelson and Liddle. 'New Labour's enemies are the irresponsible who fall down on their obligations' (cited Deacon 1996: 68). The moral reconstruction of those who are seen to flout these values, according to Frank Field, New Labour's short-lived Minister for Welfare Reform, is now the purpose of welfare:

> One of welfare's roles is to reward and to punish . . . As Christian morality becomes unsustainable without being recharged in each generation by waves of new Christian believers, so societies must seek different ways of affirming right and wrong conduct. Welfare has such a role.
>
> (Field 1996: 111)

In contrast to the new right, then, state welfare is seen as having a legitimate role in the armoury of institutions and practices through which a particular social order is maintained. Thus Tony Blair in his Foreword to the government's 1998 paper on the reform of welfare (*New Ambitions for Our Country: A New Contract for Welfare*) argued that 'it describes a third way: not dismantling welfare, nor keeping it unreformed, but reforming it on the basis of a new contract between citizen and state' (Department of Social Security 1998: v).

What Anna Coote called 'wild optimism about the capacity of public policy to influence patterns of human behaviour' (*Independent* 3 July 1995) lies at the heart of New Labour's social policies. The power of the state is to be used to create 'the basis of this modern civic society . . . an ethic of mutual responsibility or duty. It is something for something. A society where we play by the rules. You only take out if you put in. That's the bargain' (Blair 1997b). It is a social contract between individual citizens and the state in which individuals have obligations that the state is willing to assist in, principally the obligation to work and to contribute. Those who do not play by the rules are seen to have broken this contract, and are thus open to sanction: 'those individuals who wish to buck the system and oppose the verities of civilised life should not be encouraged' (Field 1996: 9). Welfare is thus moved back to the centre stage of politics, not as a means of promoting equality or overcoming the failures and deficiencies of the market, but as an instrument for forging public morality. The philosophy of communitarianism that has heavily influenced New Labour's thinking posits, according to Anna Coote, that 'humans don't need equality of opportunity or free choice so much as a sense of belonging and a clear set of rules' and as such has 'special appeal to New Labour in that it offers an intellectual security blanket, a philosophical agenda which appears to justify a shift towards civil authoritarianism' (*Independent* 3 July 1995).

## Embracing capitalism

In the third way capitalism is not challenged; rather it is embraced. New Labour's acceptance of the market differs little from that of the new right, echoing its predecessor's claim that 'there is no alternative'. As the government's report on the modernisation of Britain's tax and benefit system argued: 'There are powerful trends in society and in the global economy which, if we respond effectively to them, can be engines of prosperity and higher living standards. Resisting the challenges they pose is not a viable option' (HM Treasury 1997: 15).

The global market is seen as the final, and unchallengeable, arbiter in economic – and ultimately in social – life. But the market is not only accepted as setting the agenda and imposing constraints which national governments are powerless to resist. It is also embraced as the main provider. Like the Tories, New Labour accepts a market in state provision. Not only is the privatisation of former state industries and services left unchanged, and the encroachment of market forces and values into remaining state provision unchallenged, but these things are actively encouraged. In everything from education and health action zones to the extension of the Private Finance Initiative and proposals for pensions, private capital is seen as having a central role to play.

But a market system does not only entail the buying and selling of commodities, whether these be motor cars, hospital care or education. It also, centrally, depends on the buying and selling of human labour. The inequalities inherent in this labour market, and the enrichment of a minority which it produces, are equally accepted. 'This modern world offers rich rewards to some,' argues Peter Mandelson. 'Where these are the results of genuine initiative and creative dynamism, New Labour has no quarrel' (Mandelson 1997: 6). For those who do not succeed New Labour promises that the market will be 'fair'.

To the extent that market outcomes are seen as 'unfair' and inequitable, New Labour's quarrel is not with the market system itself – according to Labour's 1992 manifesto 'modern government has a strategic role, not to replace the market but to ensure that markets work properly' (cited N. Thompson 1996: 45). Where these do not work, the explanation is often found in the backwardness and short-termism of at least sections of British capitalism, as well as of state policy itself, and their failures to take advantage of the opportunities which global capitalism provides. According to this analysis, the problems facing British society, of unemployment or social exclusion, are not the product of market forces, themselves beyond challenge, but the consequence of the unpreparedness of British institutions to meet the market's requirements. These requirements are, in the context of the high-tech global capitalism that is now seen to rule the world, the need for flexibility, adaptability and transferable skills. According to Tony Blair:

> At the close of the twentieth century the decline of old industries and the shift to an economy based on knowledge and skills has given rise to a new class: a workless class . . . Today the greatest challenge to any democratic government is to refashion our institutions to bring this new workless class back into society and into useful work.
>
> (Blair 1997b: 7)

Thus the demand for 'education, education, education' as the Prime Minister's three over-riding objectives: a computer in every classroom, linked to the global information superhighway, producing a new generation of technologically skilled and flexible workers poised to attract the attention, investment and jobs of mobile global capital. As Gordon Brown has put it, 'in the modern global economy, where capital, raw materials and technology are internationally mobile and tradeable world-wide, it is people – their education and skills – that are necessarily the most important determinants of economic growth' (cited N. Thompson 1996: 41).

Low wages and unemployment are thus seen as problems of supply rather than demand. It is not so much that the market has failed to provide sufficient and well-paying jobs as that British workers, and the unemployed in particular, lack the skills and adaptability to attract them. It is the shortcomings of the unemployed – whether in terms of their wrong geographical location, their lack of suitable education and training or their attitudes towards work – that are the focus of government attention. As the government's 1998 paper on welfare reform (Department of Social Security 1998) makes clear, it is these 'barriers to work' that are the problem, rather than the lack of work itself or the need for job creation: both issues on which the document is conspicuously silent.

The task of government then is to prepare people for the new employment market of the twenty-first century. It is, in the language of the US workfare programmes that now has come to dominate British policy, to get people 'job ready' (Department of Social Security 1998: 25). It is emphatically not to provide the unemployed with work. As the Chancellor of the Exchequer has made clear, it is 'employment opportunity' rather than the guarantee of a job that is to be 'the modern definition of full employment for the twenty-first century' (HM Treasury 1997: 3). In this way New Labour marks a further continuity with its new-right predecessors: the role of the state, albeit enlarged in form and scope, is to act as a facilitator of the market rather than its alternative.

For New Labour this approach is to be achieved through 'partnership'. It is, however, a partnership with big business and few people else. Just as New Labour has transformed the internal workings of the Labour Party, reducing the effective voice of the trade unions and other institutions of the labour movement in the framing of policy, so it has looked to business leaders to chair reviews, assist and advise. One such example was the appointment by the government of Martin Taylor, Chief Executive of Barclays plc, to review the interaction of the tax and benefit systems and its impact on work incentives (his recommendations were incorporated into the goverment's budget in 1998 (HM Treasury 1998)); another was the appointment of Sir Peter Davies, Chief Executive of the Prudential insurance and finance company, to chair the government's task force on its welfare-to-work programme. As Thompson has argued:

> While in the 1950s and 1960s the crucial relationship in the corporate triangle was between the government and the trade union movement – particularly when Labour was in power – now, with international competitiveness the overriding goal, the crucial relationship is clearly seen as that between the Government, the City and the CBI.
>
> (N. Thompson 1996: 44)

These links are also made at a personal level. New Labour's 'friends' are, in large measure at least, different from those that Margaret Thatcher entertained. From the point of view of the British establishment, Thatcher was, and largely remained, an outsider. The daughter of a grocer, a woman, and a scientist by education and training, although married to a wealthy businessman, she never really fitted. Her popular appeal was to the forces of reaction: to the petit bourgeoisie of small businesses that felt themselves squeezed between an over-powerful state and its restrictions and regulations on the one hand, and an over-powerful trade-union movement and workforce on the other. It was an appeal to the forces of racism and xenophobia, and to those who wished to see the reinstitution of the power of the patri- archal family. It was, for all its attempts to modernise British society, essentially backward-looking. While she did her job – and from the point of view of big business she did it mostly well, significantly weak- ening organised labour and decisively shifting the balance of power and wealth in favour of capital and the rich – she was tolerated. When Thatcherism had run its course – when, for example, her nationalistic fervour threatened the future participation of British capital in an expanding European market, or her dogmatic pursuit of policies such as the Poll Tax threatened widespread civil resistance and revolt – she was abandoned. New Labour, on the other hand, presents itself as for- ward-looking, European rather than narrowly English, accepting of the changed position of women, obsessed with computers, with the modern: in a word, 'New'. Although Blair (a lawyer, and like his US counterpart, the husband of a lawyer) similarly originates from outside the British establishment – perhaps a necessary condition for anyone seeking to confront its historic backwardness – he has allied himself to what is seen as its leading edge. His friends come from the charmed cir- cles of London's professional, business and cultural elite: the world of multi-millionaire businessmen such as Richard Branson, of pop stars, the fashionable and the chic. It is an orientation not lost on the British public, 58 per cent of whom in one opinion poll considered that he 'spent too much time with the bosses, and not enough with ordinary people' (*Observer* 4 October 1998).

In political terms, New Labour's success in wresting parliamentary power from the new right has been described by David Marquand as the result of 'a remarkable coalition . . . No left-of-centre leader since the First World War has achieved anything comparable.'

> Blair has detached crucial elements of the Thatcher coalition from the Conservative Party, and enrolled them under his own banner . . . To put it in human terms, the coalition extends from John Prescott to Howard Davies, from Congress House to the CBI, from the pubs and clubs of Essex man to the senior common rooms of Oxford and Cambridge. But there is a conspicuous absentee. Except by proxy, it does not include the dispossessed of the inner cities. If they vote at all, they vote Labour. But New Labour does not need their votes, or at any rate thinks it does not need them. And so they are marginalised politically as well as socially.
>
> (Marquand 1997: 337)

In the meantime the rich are assured of their safety and prosperity. Sealed off from the world of the majority by security screens, guards, fences, on foreign islands or mansions in the countryside, they do not, in general, look willing to surrender the surplus wealth transferred to them through eighteen years of give-backs, still less to allow anyone to threaten the bedrock on which it stands. Nor does the government demand it. Instead it promises not to increase taxes. Class divisions in the meantime continue to become wider and more entrenched. Although women in general have made substantial advances, in income and employment the gulf between rich and poor women has widened. Inequalities of pay are the highest ever recorded, work is more polarised, the education, health and social gulf yawns, and the forces creating mass unemployment and poverty continue to operate. But new Labour has no programme, not even policies, for dealing with this.

Instead it looks to Middle England. It is a middle that is shrinking.

## The appeal of Middle England

As in the United States, the dramatic polarisation of income that characterised the 1980s has squeezed the numbers of those in the middle. At the same time, economic recession, particularly in the early 1990s, exposed Middle England to a taste of the insecurity – the threat of redundancy and unemployment amongst professionals and managers – that had previously largely been confined to working-class life. During the early 1990s this phenomenon became an increasing focus of media attention and political concern. As Michael Portillo, the Conservative Employment Secretary, noted in a speech to a Management of Change conference in London: 'Insecurity is felt by the middle classes as rarely before. Middle managers have been particularly hard hit' (*Guardian* 23 February 1995). In this context politicians of both political parties shifted their ground of appeal. As David Marquand argued, 'once politicians were peddlers of hope. Now they peddle security'. John Major's 'strangulated English nationalism' and Tony Blair's ethical socialism

> are all examples of a new politics of reassurance. For, as the global economy spins out of control and a rising tide of casualisation and insecurity laps around the middle class as well as the dispossessed, fear of the future diffuses all industrialised societies.
>
> (*Guardian* 3 February 1995)

What was increasingly argued, and what came to be a central plank of New Labour's successful election strategy, was that Middle England held the key to electoral victory. Just as President Clinton's New Democrats could take for granted a bedrock of support from amongst the poor, or at least their abstention from a political process in which they have in increasing numbers refused to vote, so too New Labour sought to woo the more affluent. But in appealing to Middle England, the appeal was to be to their sense of insecurity and their fears. These fears were not only about job insecurity, or the problems of negative equity that hit many, including affluent, homeowners who in a declining property market found themselves owing more to mortgage lenders than the value of their property. It was also a fear of social breakdown and disintegration, and in particular of the threat of crime that was attached to the so-called 'underclass'. Such fears are a potentially powerful combination for a reactionary politics. As Michael Portillo observed, 'insecurity . . . can bring a sense of resentment' (*Guardian* 23 February 1995), and resentment can readily fuel a search for scapegoats.

In this situation, promises to deal with 'the problem of welfare' carry an important resonance. As Tony Blair put it:

> Comfortable Britain now knows not just its own forms of insecurity and difficulty . . . It also knows the price it pays for economic and social breakdown in the poorest parts of Britain. There is a case not just in moral terms but in enlightened self interest to act to tackle what we all know exists – an underclass of people cut off from society's mainstream, without any sense of shared purpose.
>
> (Blair 1997b: 6)

New Labour may distinguish itself from its predecessors in terms of its willingness to use the resources of the state, and substantial public money, to tackle what it sees as the 'problem of the underclass', but its perception of the problem and its ultimate solution remain little changed. 'Our ambition is nothing less than a change of culture amongst benefit claimants, employers and public servants,' and foremost in this is the need to change a welfare system that 'chains people to a life of dependency' (Department of Social Security 1998: 24). The government's analysis of what it sees as the 'three fundamental problems' of welfare – the fact that, despite increasing expenditure, social exclusion has continued to grow, that the existing system traps people on welfare, and that it is open to and invites fraud and abuse – has nothing to say about the inadequacy of benefit levels or the fundamental causes of poverty. Rather it is 'welfare dependency' that remains the centre of the problem, and the solution 'to rebuild the welfare state around work' (Department of Social Security 1998: 23).

To present welfare as the problem is of course simpler and easier than a fundamental reorganisation of the economy or a critique of capitalism. As Anna Coote argued:

> Voters are worried, chiefly, about income and jobs, crime and family breakdown. On the first two, the success of Labour's policies will depend conspicuously on the health of the economy, for which the party cannot plan with any certainty. Crime and the family offer more scope for a show of strength. This is not because success is any more likely – it is not – but because measures can be adopted without any reference to the state of the economy.
>
> (*Independent* 3 July 1995)

Welfare – or at least benefits and other provisions for the poor – is thus an easy target. But at the same time, and with a middle class that feels itself squeezed and embattled, it offers the dangerous prospect of appealing to policies of greater discipline and control. As the *Independent* warned in an editorial in 1995:

> Social insecurity and fear of crime are fertile ground for a more authoritarian approach. Both here and in the US anti-crime measures are backed not only by the masses but also by a once sceptical liberal intelligentsia, which tends towards an increasingly pragmatic, pick'n'mix approach to new social controls . . . These events should worry us.
>
> (*Independent* 25 April 1995)

The shift in Labour Party thinking was taken up by Roy Hattersley, the former 'moderate' Labour politician who, since the election of New Labour, has turned into one of its most persistent critics. Writing after Harriet Harman, the Secretary of State for Social Security, criticised social-security benefits as 'handouts to the poor', he noted:

> Too often the new policies have an ugly undertone of resentment – an audible if unspoken question. How dare the certainly feeble and probably corrupt welfare recipients live on £80 a week at the expense of prosperous Britain? Increasingly the poor are being blamed for their poverty.
>
> (*Guardian* 2 April 1998).

In this context also the problem of poverty is eclipsed in New Labour's vocabulary of social exclusion. Less pejorative than the concept of 'the underclass', and more ready to consider the range of processes through which poor people are marginalised, social exclusion nevertheless remains a fundamentally conservative concept. As Ruth Levitas (1996) has argued, it stems from a continental European, and especially French, tradition and conception of social order in which social solidarity and cohesiveness is threatened by the collapse of those institutions – most notably the labour market – which are seen to bind societies together. The primary aim of social inclusion and cohesion is therefore to bind the excluded back into the labour market as a solution to the problem. That this may result in their continuing poverty is conveniently overlooked, since it is their exclusion (whether self-imposed or structural) that is the problem rather than their poverty.

So the issue of poverty slips off the political agenda, as does the need to address the adequacy of financial support for the poor. 'Those in danger of dropping off the ladder of opportunity', argued Peter Mandelson, 'will not have their long-term problems addressed by an extra pound a week on their benefit' (Mandelson 1997: 7). Certainly they won't, but New Labour goes further to argue that increasing benefit levels will only exacerbate the problem. Referring to state spending on benefits as a 'pernicious combination of profligacy and neglect', Tony Blair went on to argue: 'governments can all too easily institutionalise poverty rather than solving it. They give money out not because it is the right thing to do but because it is the easy thing to do' (Blair 1997b). So the need for 'hard' choices and 'tough' decisions – hard and tough if not for those who take them, then at least for those who bear the consequences.

## Born in the USA

When they are not looking to Middle England, Labour ministers, their advisers and spin-doctors can be seen looking to the USA. Models of the US economy, with its creation of 46.8 million new jobs since 1950, have been looked to with envy by western leaders keen to cut unemployment and reduce spending on social security. On the surface it is a story of considerable success. As one Australian commentator wryly reported, 'In the booming US economy, where unemployment is at a 25-year low, crack addicts have jobs, alcoholics have jobs, and single mothers of new-born babies have jobs . . . The atmosphere is electric' (*Sydney Morning Herald* 28 December 1997). In part this is a consequence of and is reinforced by America's welfare-to-work programme that has taken shape since the early 1990s. Like the welfare-to-work strategy that was subsequently to form the centrepiece of New Labour's welfare reforms, this programme is a mixture of drastic changes in the benefit system, coupled with mandatory job placement counselling and directed programmes to push the poor into employment.

In 1996 President Clinton fulfilled his promise to 'end welfare as we know it' by signing the Republican Party's Personal Responsibility and Work Opportunity Reconciliation Act. This Act abolished America's principal social-assistance programme, Aid to Families with Dependent Children (AFDC), and replaced it with a scheme revealingly entitled Temporary Assistance for Needy Families (TANF). At a stroke this ended automatic entitlement to cash benefits for some of the poorest of American citizens and their children. It also imposed a two-year time limit, rising to a five-year total lifetime limit on those receiving the new benefit.

Clinton's decision to support the Republican legislation was hugely symbolic. AFDC had long been a target of the American right, who argued that its support of single mothers, and of black single mothers in particular, was responsible for the creation of a dependency culture and the growth of America's 'underclass'. The ending of AFDC by a supposedly liberal Democratic president was therefore widely interpreted as signifying the acceptance of the new-right racial and moral agenda within the political mainstream. As with many measures which impact most on the poorest, this moral agenda was considerably more important than the prospect of any financial savings that might be made. Indeed, for those dependent on it, the value of benefits had already seriously declined: in 1970 the average benefit paid for a family of four was $799 a month; by 1992 it had fallen to $435 (Mercier 1994). Although the total cost of AFDC was $24 billion, this was the equivalent of the interest paid to the government's creditors every six weeks, or the amount of money consumed by the Pentagon every four (ibid.).

Unlike Britain, where a national system of poor relief, successively renamed National Assistance, Supplementary Benefit and now Income Support, provides cash benefits to a range of people in extreme poverty so long as they are not in full-time employment, the USA has never established a national universal system of means-tested assistance. In part this reflects the unwillingness of individual states to surrender their rights to decide whether relief should be given, to whom and under what circumstances, and to use public assistance – or its absence – to reinforce the operation of the differing labour markets that make up the US economy. This opposition to any national or federal programme of relief has throughout the twentieth century been most evident in the southern states of the USA, whose reliance on the low-paid labour of black Americans has, since the abolition of slavery, encouraged a hostility towards any relief system that could be seen to interfere with the incentive to work. It also reflects the historic emphasis in the USA on corporate rather than state welfare, with the result that most workers look where they can to their employers for the provision of health insurance and other benefits. The lack of a national system has meant that in general the unemployed have only had individual state, local or charitable assistance to turn to, where this exists at all.

The absence of a national system of relief was severely challenged in the depression of the 1930s, out of the political turmoil of which the New Deal was to create a federal structure of provision for certain groups. Foremost in this was a system of retirement pensions based on compulsory insurance for those in work, although, with the exception of temporary relief work, little was done for the working-aged unemployed. AFDC was similarly to emerge as a federal programme out of the New Deal. Building on a variety of schemes that individual states had adopted to provide aid for the children of widows and deserted mothers, it created a federal subsidy, in return for which those states which adopted it were required to follow certain common rules of entitlement. These earlier schemes had operated on an extremely ambivalent view that varied widely between states on who had responsibility for the support of dependent children. In general while widows with children were seen as deserving of help, unmarried mothers were expected to work, and provision mirrored the highly racialised nature of American politics and economy. Thus in 1932 82 per cent of recipients were widows, and 96 per cent of families assisted were white (Handler and Hasenfeld 1991: 70).

The introduction of AFDC as a federal programme typically failed to challenge these practices. Individual states retained considerable leeway (both officially and unofficially) to impose restrictions and exclusions, and were allowed to set their own levels of benefit. Even at the time of its abolition, average payments to a family of three, for example, ranged from $900 a month in Alaska to $130 a month in Mississippi (House of Commons Select Committee on Social Security 1998: Appendix 4, 1).

It was not until the 1960s, following the mass migration of black workers from the southern states to the industrial north, and in the face of mounting poverty and urban unrest that followed, that AFDC was expanded into a mass programme of assistance (Piven and Cloward 1993). Although changes were then introduced allowing benefit to be paid to unemployed couples with children, as well as single parents, few states took up this option and AFDC remained the major benefit payable to single mothers with children, who by the time of its abolition made up 90 per cent of claimants.

Temporary Assistance for Needy Families retained a federal subsidy to individual state expenditures, but in order to qualify for federal money states were required to move 25 per cent of welfare recipients (and 75 per cent of two-parent recipients) off welfare and into work within the first year, rising to 30 per cent (and 90 per cent of two-parent families) the following year and 50 per cent within five years. Anyone refusing or failing to find work within the time limits is liable to loss of benefits, including not only TANF but also food stamps and access to medical care under the federal Medicaid system. Within this framework individual states were given further powers to impose stricter time limits, to require mothers of children aged three months or over to find work, permanently to exclude anyone with a drug-related offence from claiming cash benefits or food stamps, to end benefits to unmarried teenage mothers (whom the law required to live with their parents or other 'responsible adults') and to deny additional benefits to anyone having a baby while in receipt of benefit. A further $100 million was allocated as an incentive to states that reduced illegitimate births and the number of abortions.

The introduction of the new welfare regime itself came in the wake of experiments that from the early 1990s had given individual states waivers from national federal AFDC regulations which allowed them to make the payment of benefit dependent on the effort to find work. One such early experiment, hailed by the Labour Party in Britain as one of 'the best international examples' of the new 'more proactive' approach to welfare (Labour Party n.d.: 2), was introduced in California under the Greater Avenues for Independence (GAIN) programme in the early 1990s. The implementation of this in Riverside County, east of Los Angeles, was the subject of a detailed study by Jamie Peck. According to this study Riverside is a prime example of the 'work first' approach to welfare reform, in which getting lone mothers into jobs takes priority over everything else, including training or adequate arrangements for the provision of childcare. In Peck's view the programme 'sets out deliberately to destabilise the experience of welfare receipt, propelling its "clients" into low-wage work with the minimum of delay, the minimum of cost and the minimum of support' (Peck 1996: 2). Based on the application of intense pressure on AFDC claimants to enter the labour market through whatever jobs were available, it was summed up quite simply by the Director of Welfare for Riverside:

It is not optional. You don't have the luxury, if you're a welfare recipient, to stay home. In fact, we insist that you come here . . . but if they don't even come and show up, we will cheerfully reduce their welfare.

(cited Peck 1996: 5)

The task of officials, themselves motivated and rewarded on the basis of performance contracts, is to get claimants 'job ready' and into work. As one manager explained:

> Job ready doesn't mean that they are trained to do something, it means they are ready to work . . . This is the basic problem that we're talking about with low-income, welfare-type people . . . it's the attitude that has to be overcome. And the way we've gone about doing that is by constant pressure, relentlessly applied. Until they get a job, and they hold a job. Or they leave the area.

(cited Peck 1996: 7)

With no call for specific job training, the emphasis is on attitude and behaviour. Claimants are issued with a set of 'Job Club Rules', including 'be on time . . . dress for success . . . no criticisms'. Intensive case management is used to supervise and constantly to reinforce the search for work, and the overwhelming message of the programme is that reliance on benefit is temporary, while any job is a good job. As Peck concludes, in the context of a labour market that is becoming increasingly polarised, and in which wages for those at the bottom are falling considerably,

> The Riverside model represents a form of economic conscription, a means of enforcing work and its associated disciplines in the context of systemic labor market failure. Here it is work itself, rather than just the work ethic, which is failing, as the problems of falling wages and insecure employment further erode the capillary processes which have traditionally operated to draw the poor into the bottom of the labor market. The brutal 'solution' represented by the Riverside approach is to intensify the 'push' from welfare into work, a classic supply-side strategy. And the Riverside philosophy makes abundantly clear, the imperative is to accept the jobs, working conditions and wages that happen to be on offer; in other words, to accommodate the labor supply to the prevailing local conditions of labor demand.

(Peck 1996: 13)

Riverside represents the most extreme example of the 'jobs first' approach to workfare under the Californian GAIN programme, although it has drawn increasing attention from and imitation by a growing number of states eager to replicate its apparent 'success' and the cheapness of its operation (Peck 1998). Elsewhere some states have given greater attention to the need for support and training to enable people to enter the labour market, although, and especially since the introduction of TANF, the pressure remains to get claimants into jobs. In Wisconsin, trailed internationally as an example of 'success' in reducing the number of people on welfare, experiments were begun in 1993, culminating in the fully fledged Wisconsin Works Programme that replaced AFDC in 1997. According to the House of Commons Select Committee on Social Security, which paid an intensive visit to the USA in 1997 in order to investigate such schemes, its purpose is 'to rebuild the connection between work and income and help families achieve self-sufficiency. The programme aims to encourage family support systems and parental responsibility, and to reinforce behaviour that leads to independence' (House of Commons Select Committee on Social Security 1998: Appendix 2, 1).

Under the Wisconsin Works Programme, which bears remarkable similarity to the scheme later introduced nationally in Britain, participants are allocated to a Financial and Employment Planner, whose task is to secure one of four options in descending order of preference: unsubsidised employment, subsidised work with an employer for up to six months at the minimum wage, a community-service job, or work training and education. As the Select Committee reported,

> Although the numbers on welfare have been reduced, expenditure on welfare programmes has not fallen by the same proportion. Indeed, far more is being spent per head on the existing caseload. Costs of supporting people in work, including subsidies for child care, transport and health care have risen.
>
> (House of Commons Select Committee on Social Security 1998: 3)

Yet as its report went on, 'If welfare reform is not concerned with reducing public expenditure, then what is its purpose? In Wisconsin the purpose is clear: to move all people capable of work from welfare into work' (ibid.). The message was unambiguous:

> Welfare claimants had to believe that they faced a life without benefit entitlement in order to concentrate their minds and ensure that they made sufficient efforts to leave welfare of their own volition . . .

to change and challenge aspects of a dependency culture, tough and frightening messages were believed to be necessary.

(House of Commons Select Committee on
Social Security 1998: 5)

The consequences of this 'tough message' were, however, less well known. Between 1994 and the end of 1997 the number of people claiming welfare fell from 14 million to 10.5 million. Yet as the Chair of the White House Council of Economic Advisers admitted, 'we have no way of knowing what happened to those who left the rolls. The question is "are we pushing more people into poverty by revamping welfare programs?" We just don't know until there is more research' (*Observer* 1 June 1997). Yet despite the apparent lack of research, the programme of 'welfare reform' goes on, 'submerged in the general desire for the State to deliver its tough message' (House of Commons Select Committee on Social Security 1998: 3). The Social Security Select Committee appeared worried by this lack of knowledge of the consequences of the state's actions, although somewhat easily assuaged by reassurances given:

We repeatedly asked whether it was possible that families with children would be allowed to become destitute in such an affluent society. The answer from virtually all concerned was that nobody knew what was going to happen, although there was an underlying belief that children would not be left to starve, if necessary by changing the laws again. In the meantime it was the message sent out by the welfare changes that was considered important.

(House of Commons Select Committee on
Social Security 1998: 5)

This message is of course not meant only, or perhaps even primarily, for those who already depend on welfare. The 'tough' messages of the social-security system have always been seen as having a far wider applicability, since, as the British National Assistance Board put it in its annual report in 1961, they 'also serve as a deterrent to others who might be tempted to follow the same course of idleness at the public expense' (National Assistance Board 1961: 36). Whether the purpose is to persuade the working poor to accept their lot or to construct particular forms of sexual and social morality, what happens to those who are dependent on the welfare system reverberates across the whole working population. Thus according to Mickey Kaus, a leading US advocate of workfare:

What's most important is not whether sweeping streets or cleaning buildings helps Betsy Smith, single teenage parent and high school dropout, learn skills that will help her find a private sector job. It is whether the prospect of sweeping streets and cleaning buildings for a welfare grant will deter Betsy Smith from having the illegitimate child that drops her out of school and onto welfare in the first place – or, failing that, whether the *sight* of Betsy Smith sweeping streets after having her illegitimate child will discourage her younger sisters and neighbors from doing as she did.

(cited Peck 1996: 11)

While there may have been little research into the fate of those pushed off the welfare rolls who failed to find a job – although it is possible that any consequent increase in crime or the turning of destitute women to prostitution would merely reinforce the image of 'the underclass' and the demand for ever more 'tough' measures – those who do find work face a low-paid and insecure future. As the senior Republican on the US welfare subcommittee of the Ways and Means Committee saw it, 'we can expect a great deal of worn rhetoric in the coming welfare debate about education for "good jobs". But the simple truth is that most welfare mothers will start out working at places like 7-Eleven or McDonald's. And what's wrong with that? Millions of Americans work for $5 an hour' (cited Mercier 1994).

Analysis by the Wisconsin Department of Workforce Development of the 42,000 jobs held by single parents who were on AFDC in one county in 1995 showed that they were concentrated in temp agencies (30 per cent), retail trades (23 per cent) and hotels, auto, business and personal services (13 per cent): all sectors 'least likely to provide sustained full-time employment' (Pawasarat 1998). Even non-temporary jobs were concentrated in a limited number of businesses, with eating and drinking establishments, nursing homes and department stores heading the list. Most of the jobs themselves were only of a very temporary nature: 75 per cent of mothers who entered the labour force were no longer employed six months later, and while only 14 per cent of jobs paid full-time wages, a mere 4 per cent paid a wage sufficient to support a family (ibid.).

This experience has since been repeated widely as federal requirements have forced even reluctant states to get single mothers off welfare and into work. As one welfare-to-work participant told an Australian reporter, 'getting a job is easy, it's getting the pay you want that's hard' (*Sydney Morning Herald* 28 December 1997). The same reporter went on:

America has put its underclass to work. Virtually everyone not incarcerated – and there are 1.7 million of those – can get a job. But the workers are exhausted. They are suffering from too much work – 12-hour shifts, seven-day weeks, 60-hour weeks. Compulsory overtime is common. Mothers drag infants on a succession of early-morning buses for the sake of a minimum-wage job . . . That's the underside of the US economic miracle – an army of worn-out, exploited working poor.

(ibid.)

## From welfare to work

The New Labour government is obsessed by work. Visiting a local Benefits Agency office two days after her appointment as Social Security Secretary, Harriet Harman argued that 'the best form of welfare for people of working age is work' (Department of Social Security Press Release, 6 May 1997). Since then the view that 'work is the best form of welfare' has settled into a mantra for New Labour policy towards the young, the disabled, the unemployed and single mothers, reiterated at every opportunity by most members of the cabinet. Work is promoted as the solution to a whole range of social issues and 'problems', with an apparent total amnesia of the damage that work has done to many people.

In his first public speech after becoming Prime Minister, Tony Blair declared that 'this will be the Welfare to Work government' (Blair 1997b: 9). Taking up the strands of the previous government's hesitant moves to adopt a national workfare scheme, the Prime Minister established an advisory task force chaired by Sir Peter Davies, Chief Executive of the Prudential insurance and financial company. By the time of the government's first budget in the autumn, a welfare-to-work scheme called the 'New Deal' for the young long-term unemployed, although already widely trailed, was formally announced: its structure bearing a remarkable similarity to that adopted in Wisconsin. This was to be implemented in a number of 'pilot' areas from January 1998, and three months later (with little apparent opportunity for evaluation of the pilots) applied nationally.

Britain's welfare-to-work programme mirrors in lots of ways its US parent. The social-security changes were, for New Labour, already in place, bequeathed by its predecessor in the form of the 1996 Jobseeker's Act. Although Labour had condemned this in opposition, once in government little was changed. The JSA, with its 'sanctions on the work-shy', was transported intact to underpin the operation of the New Deal.

In the absence of a federal structure of state government, New Labour's welfare-to-work programme has been devolved not to local authorities but to a range of new 'partnership' bodies, operating on central government's behalf. Although employers dominate these bodies, they have generally been reluctant to take part. Following the government's announcement that the majority of New Deal placements would offer long-term unemployed young people subsidised work with a private employer, estimates were soon revised down of the number of jobs likely to be available in the private sector as firms stood their distance. That many employers saw the New Deal as a form of philanthropy, rather than the business opportunity they had been waiting for, is not surprising. Few employers, at least amongst the big battalions of industry, are interested in employing workers they wouldn't employ otherwise, especially when they might turn out to be reluctant recruits from the long-term unemployed. The financial carrot of a £60 a week subsidy from government is of little interest to those firms at the leading edge of economic growth, and likely to be financially attractive only to those who pay such low wages that it makes a difference. After considerable pressure from government, however, the big battalions of industry were eventually persuaded to move publicly to the government's support, although only after securing the introduction of a screening process or 'gateway' that would weed out undesirable employees (*Financial Times* 27 August 1997), and the New Deal was launched in a £10 million advertising spree.

The New Deal for the young unemployed requires those out of work for six months or more to enter a screening process or 'Gateway' – 'an exercise in promoting job-readiness' (Department of Social Security 1998: 25) – from where they are directed into one of four options. These options are paid work with a subsidised employer, or a continuation of benefit in return for work in the voluntary sector or on an environmental task force, or training. 'There will', argued the Prime Minister, 'be no fifth option of an inactive life on benefit' (Blair 1997b). Fit young people who refuse to participate in one of the four options have all their benefit cut.

For single mothers the 'New Deal for Lone Parents' introduced alongside that for the young unemployed places less emphasis on compulsion. Instead mothers are 'invited' to interview to discuss the possible options open to them for returning to work. It remains to be seen whether persuasion will be turned to compulsion, but as Jane Lewis points out, 'even if Labour restricts its endeavours to pulling lone mothers into the labour market rather than giving them a violent push by cutting benefits wholesale, a focus on paid work does not address the equally important issue of care' (Lewis 1998: 13). As Lewis points out, while a majority of lone mothers have been shown to want to earn a decent wage, most attach more importance to the care they provide for their children. This in turn makes their involvement in the unpredictable world of the 'flexible' labour market which the majority face even more problematic. New Labour's insistence on building welfare provision around paid work fails to meet many of these problems:

> New Labour's preoccupation with stakeholding does not hold out much hope of change in this respect. Stakeholding welfare is for those in paid employment, and the aim is to get as many people into paid employment as possible . . . Lone mothers stand little chance of becoming 'equal' stakeholders because they must be both breadwinners and carers.
>
> (Lewis 1998: 11)

If the experience of the USA is anything to go by, the welfare-to-work strategy in Britain holds out little hope for the poor. At best it would seem to offer the prospect of a constant recycling of claimants through short-lived and low-paid jobs. Yet even in these terms it is a strategy that is by no means assured of success. The UK economy – like its society and its culture – is not the same as that of the USA. The capacity of American capitalism to absorb millions of extremely low-paid workers in part reflects its huge overall wealth and its vast inequalities. While the far greater disposable income of a far greater number of people may mean that they are able and willing to pay to have someone carry their groceries to the car, stand all night on security patrol outside their houses or service domestic tasks, the possibilities for an expansion of such forms of employment in Britain are much less obvious. If they are to come about, it is likely only to be as a result of yet further inequality and a massive lowering of wages.

The pauperisation of labour that the New Deal involves has a long and rather chequered history. In 1834 the Report of the Royal Commission on the Poor Laws surveyed the practice of publicly subsidised employment of the poor:

> According to this plan, the parish in general makes some agreement with a farmer to sell him the labour of one or more paupers at a certain price, and pays to the pauper, out of the parish funds, the difference between that price and the allowance which the scale,

according to the price of bread and the number of his family, awards to him . . . In other cases the parish contracts with some individual to have some work performed for him by the paupers at a given price . . . In many places the system is effected by means of an auction. In Sulgrave, Northamptonshire, the old and infirm are sold at the monthly meeting to the best bidder; at Yardley, Hastings, all the unemployed are put up to sale weekly.

(Checkland and Checkland (eds) 1974: 102)

Such practices, argued the report, encouraged employers to take on only subsidised labour, and depressed wages in general. The report also warned of the dangers of disaffection amongst those pushed into employment:

The very labourers among whom the farmer has to live, on whose merits as workmen and on whose affection as friends he ought to depend, are becoming not merely idle and ignorant and dishonest, but positively hostile; not merely unfit for his service and indifferent to his welfare, but actually desirous to injure him.

(Checkland and Checkland (eds) 1974: 145)

Caught in this pincer of claimants who see welfare to work as punishment, and a labour market in which there is little interest in employing the long-term unemployed, except in the most exploitative of situations, the government has set itself on a collision course.

## Tough choices and no alternatives

The certainty that drives the welfare-to-work programme is that, to coin a predecessor's phrase, 'there is no alternative'. 'We have to live in the world as it is,' argues Peter Mandelson, 'not as we might like it to be. And that world is a harsh, increasingly competitive world' (Mandelson 1997: 3). Global capitalism is seen as the driving force, and accepted as such. New Labour's response is simply to deliver the necessary 'flexibility'.

That this results in the continuation of poverty is not addressed. Even poverty itself is consigned to the dustbin of 'old' Labour. Frank Field, the Minister for Welfare Reform, thus described poverty as a 'national obsession' that it was now time to drop (*Telegraph* 9 June 1995), while Peter Mandelson similarly talked of achieving success 'by many different routes, not just the redistribution of cash from rich to poor which others artificially choose as their own limited definition of egalitarianism'. Instead we have what the Prime Minister describes as a 'new' phenomenon: social exclusion. As he argued in a speech at the launch of the Social Exclusion Unit in December 1997:

> It is a very modern problem, and one that is more harmful to the individual, more damaging to self-esteem, more corrosive for society as a whole, more likely to be passed down from generation to generation, than material poverty.
>
> (Blair 1997a: 4)

Poverty is not really the problem. Rather, it is those 'who have lost hope, trapped in fatalism. They are today's and tomorrow's underclass, shut out from society' (Mandelson 1997: 6). The solution to the problem is work: 'A permanently excluded underclass actually hinders flexibility rather than enhancing it. If we are to promote flexibility we must find ways of getting people off dependency and into the labour market' (Mandelson 1997: 7).

That the socially excluded are, at least in the British terminology, like the underclass, tinged with an aura of threat and menace – 'the scourge of many communities . . . young people with nothing to do [who] make life hell for other citizens' (Blair 1997b) – shows New Labour's ambivalence. It also provides justification for tighter measures of control: curfews, tagging, prosecution for 'anti-social' neighbours and those 'citizens' failing to do their duties, and incarceration for those who, presumably, are excluded the most.

What New Labour insiders refer to as 'the project' to 'modernise' British society faces severe limitations. Despite the considerable efforts of government spin-doctors and media advisers to re-brand the image of British society, to present a vision of 'Cool Britannia' as, in Tony Blair's words, 'a young country' of dynamism and change, the old ruling class remains firmly, and securely, in place, entrenched in its positions of privilege and power. It is, moreover, a country that is in economic decline, and that has been so for most of the twentieth century. No amount of image promotion is likely to change this situation. Nor is the embracing of global market forces likely to alter things for the better. Under these circumstances the prospects of alleviating the problems of chronic unemployment, poverty and inequality, let alone of creating a dynamic, open and vibrant economy, appear severely limited. If this is the case, then the danger is that what Peter Mandelson justifies as the 'tough discipline . . . necessary to break the culture of hopelessness and cynicism which a concentration of hard-core unemployment has bred in many estates throughout Britain' (cited Deacon 1996: 68) will, in the face of failure, become even tougher.

As the twentieth century draws to its close we appear – in increasing social polarisation, poverty and inequality, in the changing conditions of the labour market and in the response of state policy – to be not moving forward but returning to the nineteenth century. The gains in people's welfare achieved over a century of struggle are being swept away, and the vile maxim of the masters has returned, without disguise or embarrassment, to the centre-stage. Yet this is not the nineteenth century. Although capitalism has remained a constant, the history of the past 100 years has brought about some fundamental changes: in the position of women, in the willingness of people to challenge arbitrary authority and power, in knowledge and understanding, and in the ability of society – if not the will of its rulers – to solve what once were seen as inevitable and intractable problems. It has seen gains as well as losses, but these gains mean that the current attempt to roll back history is not conducted on the same terrain.

The present resurgence of a triumphalist capitalism does not bode well for the immediate future. Throughout the world, workers are in retreat; the advances made by women, black people, and the poor in general have been severely challenged. Defensive organisations are weakened and often in disarray, leaving people exposed to the ravages of a market system for which, we are told, there is no alternative. Hollander's comments with respect to the USA are equally applicable to Britain and indeed many other societies today:

> Throughout the United States many individuals are aware of the shifts – even the less visible ones– in our political culture, and some engage in a host of different struggles on behalf of social justice, economic equity, and authentic democracy. Unfortunately, at the present moment their critical voices are but a whisper amid the inchoate suffering of so many people. As US citizens become more anxious and insecure, the media manipulates them by focusing on sensationalist stories aimed at exacerbating real and imagined fears. Consequently the world seems ever more threatening. In response, people seem ever more willing to give up their civil rights in exchange for a paternalistic state that promises to protect them from danger. It is easy to understand how in such a climate the 1996 Antiterrorism Act readily passed into law. The irony is that the danger comes less from terrorist acts than from the terrifying economic and social conditions endemic to the neoliberal framework of late capitalism.
>
> (Hollander 1997: 231)

But this circumstantial pessimism is, for us, tempered by an historical optimism informed by the resistance over many centuries of ordinary people to oppression and injustice. The evident inhumanity of the vile maxim is also its greatest vulnerability. This is why so much effort is put into denying its existence and its consequences. It is why attempts are made to shift the blame elsewhere, and to divide the poor amongst themselves both nationally and internationally. If this book has done one thing, we hope that it has exposed this inhumanity and hypocrisy, and if it leads to one thing we hope it leads to a greater rage against a system that debases people for private profit. Too many seem to have lost their sense of anger at what is happening in our midst. Yet without anger the possibilities of fundamental social and political change will always be elusive.

# References and bibliography

Adams, W. (1953). 'Lloyd George and the labour movement.' *Past and Present* 3.

Alderson, J. (1996). 'A fair cop.' *Red Pepper* 24 (May): 11–13.

Allbeson, J. (1985). 'Seen but not heard: young people.' In S. Ward (ed.) *DHSS In Crisis*. London, Child Poverty Action Group.

Andrews, K. and J. Jacobs (1990). *Punishing the Poor: Poverty Under Thatcher*. London, Macmillan.

Anon. (1889). 'Socialism and self help.' *London Quarterly Review* 72: 241–62.

Archbishop of Canterbury's Commission on Urban Priority Areas (1985). *Faith in the City: A Call for Action by Church and Nation*. London, Church House Publishing.

Arnold, A. (1888). 'Socialism and the unemployed.' *Contemporary Review* 53: 560–71.

Atherley-Jones, L. (1893). 'Liberalism and social reform: a warning.' *The New Review* 9: 629–35.

Atkinson, A. B. (1996). 'Seeking to explain the distribution of income.' In J. Hills *New Inequalities*. Cambridge, Cambridge University Press. 19–48.

Barter, C. (1996). *Nowhere to Hide*. London: Centrepoint.

Becker, S. and G. Craig (1989). 'The fund that likes to say no.' *Social Work Today* (8 June): 13–15.

Becker, S. and R. Silburn (1990). *The New Poor Clients*. Wallington, Community Care.

Bell, L. and S. A. Webb (1992). 'The invisible art of teaching for practice.' *Social Work Education* 11(1): 28 46.

Beveridge, W. (1906). 'The problem of the unemployed.' *Sociological Papers* 3: 323–41.

—— (1942). *Social Insurance and Allied Services*. Cmnd 6404. London, HMSO.

—— (1945). *Full Employment in a Free Society*. London, George Allen and Unwin.

Beynon, H. (1983). 'False hopes and real dilemmas: the politics of the collapse in British manufacturing.' *Critique* 16: 1–22.

Blair, T. (1997a). Speech at Stockwell Park School, Lambeth, 8 December. (http://www.open.gov.uk/co/seu.more.html/speech by the prime minister)

## 204 References and bibliography

Blair, T. (1997b). Speech at the Aylesbury Estate, Southwark, 2 June. (http://www.open.gov.uk/co/seu.more.html/speech by the prime minister)

Bluestone, B. and B. Harrison (1982). *The Deindustrialization of America*. New York, Basic Books.

Booth, C. (1904). *Life and Labour of the People in London*. London, Macmillan.

Bosanquet, B. (1895). *Aspects of the Social Problem*. London, Macmillan.

Bosanquet, H. (1893). 'The industrial residuum.' *Economic Journal* 3: 600–16.

—— (1896). *The Rich and the Poor*. London, Macmillan.

Bottomley, V. (1994). *National Core Curriculum for Social Work Training*. Conservative Party News (26 February). 137/94.

Brenner, R. (1998). 'The economics of global turbulence.' *New Left Review* (229): special issue.

Brewster, R. (1992). 'The new class? Managerialism and social work education and training.' *Issues in Social Work Education* 11(2): 81–93.

Bridges, L. (1983). 'Policing the urban wasteland.' *Race and Class* 25(2): 31–48.

Brittan, S. (1976). In *Why Is Britain Becoming Harder To Govern?* London, BBC Publications.

Brosnan, P. and F. Wilkinson (1987). *Low Pay: Britain's False Economy*. London, Low Pay Unit.

Bryan, B., S. Dadzi and S. Scafe (1985). *The Heart of the Race: Black Women's Lives in Britain*. London, Virago.

Burleigh, B. (1887). 'The unemployed.' *Contemporary Review* 52: 770–80.

Byrne, D. (1994). 'Deindustrialisation and dispossession: an examination of social division in the industrial city.' *Sociology* 29(1): 95–115.

Campbell, B. (1988). *Unofficial Secrets: The Cleveland Case*. London, Virago.

—— (1993). *Goliath: Britain's Dangerous Places*. London, Methuen.

Campfens, H. (1992). 'The new reality of poverty and social work interventions.' *International Social Work* 35(2): 99–104.

Carter, B. and P. Fairbrother (1995). 'The remaking of the state middle classes.' In T. Butler and M. Savage *Social Change and the Middle Classes*. London, UCL Press. 133–47.

Chambers, R. (1994). 'Poverty and livelihoods: whose reality counts?' Paper presented to the United Nations Stockholm Roundtable on Global Change.

Checkland, S. and E. Checkland (eds) (1974). *The Poor Law Report of 1834*. Harmondsworth, Penguin.

Children's Rights Development Unit (1994). *UK Agenda for Children*. London, CRDU.

Chomsky, N. (1977). 'Trilateral's rx for crisis: governability yes, democracy no.' *Seven Days* (14 February): 10–11.

—— (1993). *Year 501: The Conquest Continues*. London, Verso.

—— (1996). 'Rollback II: "civilization" marches on.' *Z-Magazine*: (http://www.lbbs.org/zmag/articles/chom2.htm)

Christie, N. (1996). 'Crime and civilisation.' *New Internationalist* 282: 10–12.

Churchill, R. (1967). *Winston S. Churchill*. London, Heinemann.

Clarke, J. and J. Newman (1997). *The Managerial State*. London, Sage.

Coates, K. and R. Silburn (1970). *Poverty: The Forgotten Englishmen.* Harmondsworth, Penguin Books.

Cook, D. (1998). 'Between a rock and a hard place: the realities of working on the side.' *Benefits* 21: 11–15.

Cooper, S. (1985). *Observations in Supplementary Benefit Offices: The Reform of Supplementary Benefit: Working Paper C.* London, Policy Studies Institute.

Corrigan, P. (1977). 'State formation and moral regulation in nineteenth century Britain.' Unpublished PhD thesis, University of Durham.

Corrigan, P. and D. Sayer (1985). *The Great Arch: English State Formation as Cultural Revolution.* Oxford, Basil Blackwell.

Cracknell, R., T. Jarvis and W. Wilson (1996). *The Social Security Administration (Fraud) Bill.* House of Commons Research Paper 96/107. London, House of Commons Library.

Craig, G. (1988). 'Nightmare lottery of the Social Fund.' *Social Work Today* (24 November): 15–17.

—— (1998). 'The privatisation of human misery.' *Critical Social Policy* 18(1): 51–76.

Crozier, M., S. P. Huntington and J. Watanuki (1975). *The Crisis of Democracy: The Trilateral Commission Task Force Report No. 8.* New York, New York University Press.

Davidson, R. (1971). 'Sir Hubert Llewellyn-Smith and labour policy 1886–1916.' PhD Unpublished thesis, University of Cambridge.

Davies, N. (1997). *Dark Heart.* London, Chatto and Windus.

Davies, P. (1998). *This England.* London, Abacus.

Davis, A. and S. Wainwright (1996). 'Poverty work and the mental health services.' *Breakthrough* 1(1): 47–56.

Deacon, A. (1996). 'Welfare and character.' In A. Deacon *Stakeholder Welfare.* London, Institute for Economic Affairs.

Department of Employment (1988). *Labour Market Trends: June 1988.* London, HMSO.

—— (1996). *Labour Market Trends: June 1996.* London, HMSO.

Department of Health and Social Security (1986). *Reform of Social Security. Volume 2: Programme for Change.* Cmnd 9518. London, HMSO.

Department of Social Security (1998). *New Ambitions for Our Country: A New Contract for Welfare.* Cmnd 3805. London, HMSO.

de Schweinitz, K. (1947). *England's Road to Social Security: 1349–1947.* Pennsylvania, University of Pennsylvania Press.

Eaton, L. (1996). 'Poor standards.' *Community Care* (13/19 June): 10.

Eden, F. (1796). *The State of the Poor: Or, An History of the Labouring Classes in England.* Repr. London, Frank Cass, 1966.

Edgar, D. (1983). 'Bitter harvest.' *New Socialist* (September/October): 19–24.

Evason, E. and R. Woods (1995). 'Poverty, deregulation of the labour market and benefit fraud.' *Social Policy and Administration* 29(1): 40–54.

Fabian Society (1886). *The Government Organisation of Unemployed Labour.* London, Standring.

Field, F. (1996). 'Stakeholder welfare.' In A. Deacon *Stakeholder Welfare*. London, Institute of Economic Affairs.

Finn, D. and I. Murray (1995). *Unemployment and Training Rights Handbook*. London, Unemployment Unit.

Franklin, B. (1989). 'Wimps and bullies: press reporting of child abuse.' In P. Carter, T. Jeffs and M. Smith *Social Work and Social Welfare Yearbook 1*. Milton Keynes, Open University Press.

Fry, A. (1991). 'Under inspection.' *Social Work Today* (20 June): 16–17.

Gaillie, D. (1994). 'Are the unemployed an underclass? Some evidence from the social change and economic life initiative.' *Sociology* 28(3): 737–57.

George, V. and P. Wilding (1976). *Ideology and Social Welfare*. London, Routledge and Kegan Paul.

Gilbert, B. (1966). *The Evolution of National Insurance in Great Britain: The Origins of the Welfare State*. London, Michael Joseph.

Gill, S. (1980). 'The Trilateral Commission, the international economy and structural policy.' *Journal of Industrial Affairs* 7(2): 38–42.

Goldson, B. (1999). 'Youth (in)justice: contemporary developments in policy and practice.' In B. Goldson *Youth Justice: Contemporary Policy and Practice*. Aldershot, Ashgate.

Gray, A. (1998). 'New Labour – new labour discipline.' *Capital and Class* (65): 1–8.

Green, Penny (1990). *The Enemy Without: Policing and Class Consciousness in the Miners' Strike*. Milton Keynes, Open University Press.

Green, Pete (1987). 'British capitalism and the Thatcher years.' *International Socialism* 2(35): 3–70.

Gregg, P. and J. Wadsworth (1995). 'A short history of labour turnover, job tenure and job security, 1975–1993.' *Oxford Review of Economic Policy* 11(1): 73–90.

Gutzmore, C. (1983). 'Capital, "black youth" and crime.' *Race and Class* 25(2): 13–30.

Habermas, J. (1983). 'Neoconservative culture criticism in the United States and West Germany: an intellectual movement in two political cultures.' *Telos* 56 (Summer): 75–89.

Hadley, R. and R. Clough (1996). *Care in Chaos*. London, Cassell.

Hammond, J. L. and B. Hammond (1913). *The Village Labourer 1760–1832*. London, Longman Green & Co.

Handler, J. F. (1968). 'The co-ercive children's officer.' *New Society* (3 October): 485–7.

Handler, J. F. and Y. Hasenfeld (1991). *The Moral Construction of Poverty: Welfare Reform in America*. London, Sage.

Harris, C. (1991). 'Configurations of racism: the civil service, 1945–60.' *Race and Class* 33(1): 1–30.

Harris, J. (1972). *Unemployment and Politics: A Study in English Social Policy 1886–1914*. Oxford, Oxford University Press.

Harris, N. (1961). 'The decline of welfare.' *International Socialism* 7: 5–14.

Hasbach, W. (1908). *A History of the English Agricultural Labourer*. London, P. S. King.

Haughey, O. (1998). 'Lone parents and the Labour government's New Deal – welfare to work.' Unpublished MA thesis, University of Liverpool.

Heath, A. (1992). 'The attitudes of the underclass.' In D. Smith *Understanding the Underclass*. London, Policy Studies Institute.

Hernstein, R. and C. Murray (1994). *The Bell Curve: Intelligence and Class Structure in American Life*. New York, Simon and Schuster.

Hewlett, S. A. (1993). *Child Neglect in Rich Nations*. New York, UNICEF.

Hills, J. (1996). *New Inequalities: The Changing Distribution of Income and Wealth in the United Kingdom*. Cambridge, Cambridge University Press.

HM Treasury (1997). *The Modernisation of Britain's Tax and Benefit System. Number One. Employment Opportunity in a Changing Labour Market.* London, HM Treasury. (http://www.hm-treasury.gov.uk/-pub/html/docs/fpp/mtb/main.html)

—— (1998). *The Modernisation of Britain's Tax and Benefit System. Number Two. Work Incentives: A Report by Martin Taylor.* London, HM Treasury.

Hoggart, R. (1960). 'The welfare state: appearance and reality.' *Social Work* 17: 13–17.

Hollander, N. C. (1997). *Love in a Time of Hate: Liberation Psychology in Latin America*. New Brunswick, Rutgers University Press.

Hollis, P. (1973). *Class and Conflict in Nineteenth Century England*. London, Routledge and Kegan Paul.

Holman, B. (1993). *A New Deal for Social Welfare*. Oxford, Lion.

Home Office (1998). *Crime and Disorder Act 1998: Introductory Guide.* London, Home Office.

House of Commons Select Committee on Social Security (1998). *Social Security Reforms: Lessons from the United States of America. Second Report.* London, HMSO.

Howe, L. (1985). 'The "deserving" and "undeserving": practice in an urban, local social security office.' *Journal of Social Policy* 14(1): 49–72.

Irvine, E. E. (1954). 'Research into problem families.' *British Journal of Psychiatric Social Work* 9 (Spring): 24–33.

Jackson, C. and J. Pringle (1909). 'The effects of unemployment or assistance given to the unemployed since 1886.' In *Report of the Royal Commission on the Poor Laws and the Relief of Distress*, Appendix, vol. xix.

Jones, A. (1993). 'UK: Anti-racist child protection.' *Race and Class* 35(2): 75–85.

Jones, C. and T. Novak (1985). 'Welfare against the workers: benefits as a political weapon.' In H. Beynon *Digging Deeper*. London, Verso.

—— (1993). 'Social work today.' *British Journal of Social Work* 23(3): 195–212.

Jordan, B. (1988). 'Poverty, social work and the state.' In S. Becker and S. MacPherson *Public Issues Private Pain*. London, Insight.

Judis, J. B. (1983). 'The right and the wrongs of Reagan.' *The Progressive* (January): 22–7.

Kay-Shuttleworth, J. (1832). *The Moral and Physical Condition of the Working Classes*. Repr. London, Frank Cass, 1970.

Kaye, H. J. (1995). 'Why do ruling classes fear history?' *Index on Censorship* 24(3): 85–98.

Kraemer, S. and J. Roberts (1996). *The Politics of Attachment*. London, Free Association Books.

Kushnick, L. (1990). 'US: the revocation of civil rights.' *Race and Class* 32(1): 57–66.

Labour Party (n.d.). *Getting Welfare to Work: A New Vision for Social Security*. London, Labour Party.

Larochelle, C. and H. Campfens (1992). 'The structure of poverty: a challenge for the training of social workers in the North and South.' *International Social Work* 35(2): 105–19.

Lavalette, M. and J. Kennedy (1996). *Solidarity on the Waterfront*. Liverpool, Liver Press.

Levitas, R. (1986). 'Tory students and the new right.' *Youth and Policy* (16): 1–9.

—— (1996). 'The concept of social exclusion and the new Durkheimian hegemony.' *Critical Social Policy* 16(1): 5–20.

Levy, S. (1970). *Nassau W. Senior*. Newton Abbot, David and Charles.

Lewis, J. (1998). '"Work", "welfare" and lone mothers.' *Political Quarterly* 69(1): 4–13.

Llewellyn-Smith, H. (1910). 'Economic security and unemployment insurance.' *Economic Journal* 20: 513–29.

Lloyd George, D. (1911). *The People's Insurance*. London, Hodder and Stoughton.

Low Pay Unit (1994). *The New Review* November/December.

MacDonald, R. (1994). 'Fiddly jobs, undeclared work and the something for nothing society.' *Work, Employment & Society* 8(4): 507–30.

MacKay, T. (1902). 'The Poor Law and the economic order.' *Economic Review* 12: 278–88.

Macnicol, J. (1987) 'In pursuit of the underclass.' *Journal of Social Policy* 16(3): 293–318.

Mandelson, P. (1997). *Labour's Next Steps: Tackling Social Exclusion*. London, Fabian Society.

Mandelson, P. and R. Liddle (1996). *The Blair Revolution*. London, Faber and Faber.

Marable, M. (1997). *Black Liberation in Conservative America*. Boston, South End Press.

Marquand, D. (1997). 'After euphoria: the dilemmas of New Labour.' *Political Quarterly* 68(4): 335–8.

Marshall, G., S. Roberts and C. Burgoyne (1996). 'Social class and underclass in Britain and the USA.' *British Journal of Sociology* 47(1): 22–44.

Marx, K. (1968). *Selected Correspondence*. Moscow, Progress Publishers.

—— (1973). *Grundrisse*. Harmondsworth, Pelican.

—— (1974). *Capital Vol. I*. London, Lawrence and Wishart.

Massey, D. (1983). 'The new geography of jobs.' *New Society* (17 March): 416–18.

May, T. (1991). *Probation: Politics, Policy and Practice*. Milton Keynes, Open University Press.

McCarthy, M. (1989). 'Crusade against the welfare state.' *Social Work Today* (25 May): 21.

McCrate, E. and J. Smith (1998). 'When work doesn't work.' *Gender and Society* 12(1): 61–80.

McGregor, O. (1957). 'Sociology and welfare.' *Sociological Review Monograph* 4.

Mercier, R. (1994). 'Welfare reform.' *Z-Magazine* (September).

Murray, C. (1984). *Losing Ground: American Social Policy 1950–1980*. New York, Basic Books.

—— (1990). *The Emerging British Underclass*. London, Institute of Economic Affairs.

Nairne, P. (1983). 'Managing the DHSS elephant: reflections on a giant department.' *Political Quarterly* 54(3): 243–56.

NALGO (1989). *Social Work in Crisis*. London, NALGO.

National Assistance Board (1961) *Annual Report.* London, HMSO.

Novak, T. (1988). *Poverty and the State: An Historical Sociology*. Milton Keynes, Open University Press.

Novak, T. and H. Sennett (1996). 'Changing social work.' In J. Clarke *The Hitchiker's Guide to D211*. Milton Keynes, Open University. 72–8.

Office for National Statistics (1995). *Social Trends 25*. London, HMSO.

—— (1997). *Social Trends 27*. London, HMSO.

Oliver, M. and C. Barnes (1998). *Disabled People and Social Policy*. London, Longman.

Oppenheim, C. (1993). *Poverty: The Facts*. London, Child Poverty Action Group.

—— (1997) 'The growth of poverty and inequality.' In A. Walker and C. Walker *Britain Divided*. London, Child Poverty Action Group. 17–31.

Oppenheim, C. and L. Harker (1996). *Poverty: The Facts*. London, Child Poverty Action Group.

Oppenheim, J. (1987). 'Falling apart at the seams.' *Insight* (20 November): 10–11.

Pawasarat, J. (1998). 'The employer perspective: jobs held by the Milwaukee County AFDC single parent population.' In House of Commons Select Committee on Social Security, *Social Security Reforms: Lessons from the United States of America. Second Report*. London, HMSO.

Payne, J. and C. Payne (1994). 'Recession, restructuring and the fate of the unemployed: evidence in the underclass debate.' *Sociology* 28(1): 1–19.

Peck, J. (1996). 'Local discipline: workfare as labor control.' Paper presented at the conference 'The Globalisation of Production and the Regulation of Labour', University of Warwick.

—— (1998). 'Workfare in the sun: politics, representation and method in U.S. welfare-to-work strategies.' *Political Geography* 17(5): 535–66.

Pelling, H. (1968). 'The working class and the origins of the welfare state.' In H. Pelling *Popular Politics and Society in Late Victorian Britain*. London, Macmillan.

Phillips, D. (1989). 'Young people under pressure from government.' *Social Work Today* (15 June): 22-3.

Piachaud, S. (1997). 'The growth of means-testing.' In A. Walker and C. Walker *Britain Divided: The Growth of Social Exclusion in the 1980s and 1990s*. London, Child Poverty Action Group.

Pilger, J. (1998). *Hidden Agendas*. London, Vintage.

Piven, F. and R. Cloward (1993). *Regulating the Poor: The Functions of Public Welfare*. New York, Pantheon.

Poynter, J. (1969). *Society and Pauperism: English Ideas on Poor Relief 1795–1834*. London, Routledge and Kegan Paul.

Prebble, J. (1969). *The Highland Clearances*. Harmondsworth, Penguin.

Rae, J. (1890). 'State socialism and social reform.' *Contemporary Review* 58: 435–54.

Raup, E. (1996). 'Politics, race and US penal strategies.' *Soundings* 2: 153–68.

Rea, R. (1912). *Social Reform Versus Socialism*. London, Liberal Publications Department.

*Report of the Royal Commission on the Poor Laws and Relief of Distress* (1909). London, HMSO.

Richan, W. C. and A. R. Mendelsohn (1973). *Social Work: The Unloved Profession*. New York, New Viewpoints.

Roberts, J. and S. Kraemer (1996). 'Introduction: holding the thread.' In S. Kraemer and J. Roberts *The Politics of Attachment*. London, Free Association Books.

Rodgers, B. (1960). *Portrait of Social Work: A Study of Social Services in a Northern Town*. London, Oxford University Press.

Rose, D. (1992). *A Climate of Fear: The Murder of PC Blakelock and the Case of the Tottenham Three*. London, Bloomsbury.

—— (1996). *In the Name of the Law*. London, Vintage.

Rose, M. (1971) *The English Poor Law 1780–1930*. Newton Abbot, David and Charles.

Rothstein, T. (1929). *From Chartism to Labourism*. London, Martin Lawrence.

Rowlingson, K. and C. Whyley (1998). '"The right amount to the right people"? Reducing fraud, error and non-take-up of benefit.' *Benefits* 21: 7–10.

Ryan, D. (1998). 'The Thatcher government's attack on higher education in historical perspective.' *New Left Review* 227 (January/February): 3–32.

Sainsbury, R. (1998). 'Putting fraud into perspective.' *Benefits* 21: 2–6.

Satyamurti, C. (1974). 'Women's occupation and social change: the case of social work.' British Sociological Association, annual conference, unpublished paper.

Saville, J. (1957). 'The welfare state: an historical approach.' *The New Reasoner* 3, (Winter): 1–24.

Scheper-Hughes, N. (1997). 'People who get rubbished.' *New Internationalist* 295: 20–2.

Schorr, A. (1992). *The Personal Social Services: An Outsider's View*. York, Joseph Rowntree Foundation.

Scraton, P. (1984). 'The coroner's tale.' In P. Scraton and P. Gordon *Causes for Concern: British Criminal Justice on Trial*. Harmondsworth, Pelican Original.

Seabrook, J. (1998). 'Children of the market.' *Race and Class* 39(4): 37–48.

Segalman, R. and D. Marsden (1989). *Cradle to Grave*. London, Social Affairs Unit.

Selman, P. and C. Glendenning (1994/5). 'Teenage parenthood and social policy.' *Youth and Policy* 47: 39–58.

Senior, N. (1865). *Historical and Philosophical Essays*. London, Longman Green.

Shichor, D. and D. K. Sechrest (eds) (1996). *Three Strikes and You're Out*. London, Sage.

Silk, L. and M. Silk (1980). *The American Establishment*. New York, Avon Discuss Books.

Sivanandan, A. (1996). 'La trahison des clercs.' *Race and Class* 37(3): 65–70.

—— (1998). 'The making of home to the beat of a different drum.' *Race and Class* 39(3): 73–8.

Sklar, H. (1995). *Chaos or Community*? Boston, South End Press.

—— (ed.) (1980). *Trilateralism*. Boston, South End Press.

Smith, D. (ed.) (1992). *Understanding the Underclass*. London, Policy Studies Institute.

Smith, G. and R. Harris (1972). 'Ideologies of need and organisation of social work departments.' *British Journal of Social Work* 2(1): 27–45.

Smith, R. (1987). *Unemployment and Health*. Oxford, Oxford University Press.

Steinfels, P. (1979). *The Neoconservatives*. New York, Simon and Schuster.

Thane, P. (1984). 'The working class and state welfare in Britain.' *Historical Journal* 27(4): 877–900.

Thompson, A. (1996). 'A word to the wise.' *Community Care* (27 June): 14–15.

Thompson, N. (1996). 'Supply side socialism: the political economy of New Labour.' *New Left Review* (216): 37–54.

Titmuss, R. M. (1968). *Commitment to Welfare*. New York, Pantheon Books.

Townsend, P., P. Corrigan and U. Kowarzik (1987). *Poverty and Labour in London*. London, Low Pay Unit.

Trilateral Commission (1979). *Industrial Policy and the International Economy*. New York, Trilateral Commission.

Unemployment Unit (1991). *Working Brief* (November).

—— (1993). *Working Brief* (42).

—— (1994). *Working Brief* (52).

—— (1995). *Working Brief* (63).

US Bureau of Census (1994). *Press Release*: 'Median net worth of households dropped 12 percent.' (http://www.us.gov:70/00/Bureau/Pr/Subject/Income/ch94-06.txt)

Walker, A. and C. Walker (eds) (1997). *Britain Divided: The Growth of Social Exclusion in the 1980s and 1990s*. London, Child Poverty Action Group.

Walley, J. (1972). *Social Security: Another British Failure*. London, C. Knight.

Wardhaugh, J. and P. Wilding (1993). 'Towards an explanation of the corruption of care.' *Critical Social Policy* 13(1): 4–31.

Webb, S. (1890). 'The reform of the Poor Law.' *Contemporary Review* 58: 95–120.

Webb, S. and B. Webb (1929). *English Local Government*. London, Longman Green & Co.

Webster, D. (1998). 'Hard labour: can policies to tackle social exclusion work without new jobs?' *Inside Housing* (13 March).

Wilkinson, R. G. (1994). *Unfair Shares*. Ilford, Barnardo's.

—— (1996). *Unhealthy Societies*. London, Routledge.

Williams, R. (1961). *The Long Revolution*. London, Chatto and Windus.

—— (1989). *Resources of Hope*. London, Verso.

Winter, J. (1974). *Socialism and the Challenge of War*. London, Routledge.

Wolfe, A. (1980). 'Capitalism shows its face: giving up on democracy.' In H. Sklar *Trilateralism*. Boston, South End Press. 295–307.

Wolff, E. (1995). 'How the pie is sliced: America's growing concentration of wealth.' *American Prospect* 22: 58–64.

Women's Group on Public Welfare (1943). *Our Towns*. Oxford, Oxford University Press.

Wootton, B. (1944). *Social Security and the Beveridge Plan*. London, Common Wealth.

# Index